CW01583703

Changing Substance Abuse and Criminal Behavior Through Therapeutic Relationships

Debra H. Benveniste

Changing Substance Abuse and Criminal Behavior Through Therapeutic Relationships

palgrave
macmillan

Debra H. Benveniste
Dayville, Connecticut, USA

ISBN 978-1-137-53038-7 ISBN 978-1-137-53039-4 (eBook)
DOI 10.1057/978-1-137-53039-4

Library of Congress Control Number: 2016938716

© The Editor(s) (if applicable) and The Author(s) 2016
The author(s) has/have asserted their right(s) to be identified as the author(s) of this work in accordance with the Copyright, Designs and Patents Act 1988.
This work is subject to copyright. All rights are solely and exclusively licensed by the Publisher, whether the whole or part of the material is concerned, specifically the rights of translation, reprinting, reuse of illustrations, recitation, broadcasting, reproduction on microfilms or in any other physical way, and transmission or information storage and retrieval, electronic adaptation, computer software, or by similar or dissimilar methodology now known or hereafter developed.
The use of general descriptive names, registered names, trademarks, service marks, etc. in this publication does not imply, even in the absence of a specific statement, that such names are exempt from the relevant protective laws and regulations and therefore free for general use.
The publisher, the authors and the editors are safe to assume that the advice and information in this book are believed to be true and accurate at the date of publication. Neither the publisher nor the authors or the editors give a warranty, express or implied, with respect to the material contained herein or for any errors or omissions that may have been made.

Cover illustration: © Steven C. Ross

Printed on acid-free paper

This Palgrave Pivot imprint is published by Springer Nature
The registered company is Macmillan Publishers Ltd. London

Acknowledgments and Dedication

Although I am the author of this book, in many ways I have only been a conduit for others. A great many of the people who contributed to this book will have to go unnamed. I know that many of them had hoped that there was something positive about themselves that they could give to others to make up for the damage they have caused. Others are deceased and never had the chance to realize their potential in life. I have attempted to convey what was compelling, wise, and important about all of them, so that those qualities can live on in some way.

I started out in this field as a drug counselor, working without the benefit of a clinical degree. My first clients, particularly Billy, Bobby, and Jeff, patiently and thoroughly schooled me about the nature of heroin addiction. They helped me to be wise beyond my young age and lack of experience. Many of those clients succumbed to the AIDS pandemic just as it was beginning.

The Smith College School for Social Work provided me with an excellent education in psychodynamic theory and therapy. Post master's, the incarcerated clients I worked with, particularly Marc and Ron, allowed me into their internal worlds and helped me to understand the complexity of violent crime. Since then in private practice, I have worked with clients with substance abuse problems and those in secondary desistance from criminal behavior. A thank you to Terry, Jeff, and Bill, who helped me to understand the role of trauma in substance abuse.

To all of my clients who have lost hard-fought battles with their demons, may they rest in peace.

I am thankful to Simmons College School of Social Work and my doctoral committee for supporting the dissertation which produced the results used for this book. I am especially grateful to Dr Heith Copes for his wisdom and availability. A very special thanks to Sam Williams, the community advisor for the project, whose help with the pilot study was invaluable. I am very grateful to the "group of 11," my respondents who gave of their time and of themselves to share their desistance process with me. I thoroughly enjoyed meeting with them and wish them all the very best in their journeys. Thank you to Nicola Jones and Eleanor Christie at Palgrave Macmillan for their support of this work. I am grateful to Shannon Dohar for her reading of the manuscript and for her advice and suggestions. This book is dedicated to my husband, Steve, who has provided me with unfailing support and encouragement throughout all of these endeavors.

Contents

List of Figures and Tables

Figures

Tables

Part I

Overview

This book chronicles the journeys of 11 men who successfully desisted from long-term substance abuse and criminal behavior. Qualitative data derived from their interviews was analyzed to explore how relationships with significant others were utilized to facilitate their desistance. Using relational analytic theory as a framework, the author applies the data to therapy with this client population and formulates a practice model. Basic relational concepts including mutual co-construction of the therapy relationship, dissociation, and enactment provide its structure. The phases of treatment necessary to facilitate desistance including relational goals, attachment and engagement, witnessing, identification, therapeutic conflict, the capacity for internal conflict, personal agency, identity change, and meaning making are described. These concepts are applied to current agency practice.

1

Introduction

Abstract The first chapter provides an overview of the scope of the book and introduces its basic concepts and goals. Specifics of the research project which generated the interviews are discussed including special issues in analysis and presentation of the data. The author argues for the choice of psychodynamic theory to explain the data and derive a practice model. Cognitive behavioral therapy (CBT) with the substance abuser and offender populations is the current treatment of choice, yet some practice models are evolving to incorporate psychodynamic principles. Examples of treatment programs for substance abusers and offenders that integrate CBT and psychodynamic concepts are presented. The author's practice model integrating relational analytic theory, interview data, and case examples with these client populations is introduced.

This book began as a compilation of 11 men's stories of an extraordinary accomplishment: their successful desistance from substance abuse and criminal behavior. Beginning from lives defined by criminal acts including assault, robbery, theft, substance abuse, and drug dealing, they each recounted the process they underwent to desist from these activities. From childhoods ravaged by poverty, urban ghettoes, childhood trauma, and family dysfunction to adolescence which began the descent into school truancy, drug addiction, violence,

© The Editor(s) (if applicable) and The Author(s) 2016

D.H. Benveniste, *Changing Substance Abuse and Criminal Behavior Through Therapeutic Relationships*, DOI 10.1057/978-1-137-53039-4_1

and life within a criminal subculture, their early adulthoods culminated in criminal behavior, victimization, rage, addiction, incarceration, and despair.

But the typical continuation of this life course to long-term incarceration, physical debilitation, and early death stopped there. Each man came to the realization that he no longer wanted to live in this manner and began his search for a way out, a complex and multi-year process often filled with multiple treatment attempts and false starts. The desistance path they each ultimately found was facilitated by relationships with others who helped to make this life change feasible. Many were therapists, counselors, and 12 Step program sponsors.

This work utilizes results from a dissertation submitted as part of a PhD in social work. The qualitative, interview-based study completed for the dissertation explored how men who had stopped engaging in violent behavior thought about and described the role of significant relationships in their desistance process. Special emphasis was placed on the mechanisms functioning within these relationships that initiated this process as well as for the support of ongoing desistance.

Specifics of the study's rationale and methodology are located in the Appendix and at the beginning of Chap. 2. For confidentiality purposes, respondents were asked for pseudonyms that were used in all study documentation. These nicknames were retained for use in this book. Direct quotations from sources were edited to remove non-verbal utterances and reworded for clarity. However, care was taken to maintain their meaning. The consent form that study respondents signed before beginning their interviews gave permission for me to use their data for the dissertation and further research works.

At the time of the interview, study participants were living in the community (not incarcerated) and had been sober and crime-free from between several months to a decade or more, representing many different points along the desistance continuum. As the study progressed, several additional factors about the respondents became evident. Potential study participants were accessed through social service agencies providing their treatment, and 10 of 11 also had a history of serious substance abuse. All but one were actively involved in treatment for either substance abuse or mental health or for both. These factors proved crucial to the formulation of this work. Two other major aspects of life and identity presented by the respondents, HIV status and homosexuality, were not explored as part of the study or for this book.

Throughout the interview process and from a retrospective vantage point, respondents were able to piece together the aspects of their significant relationships most important to their desistance processes. Many described relationships with family members such as parents, siblings, partners, children, nieces and nephews, and grandchildren, but just as many credited treatment experiences as critical to their desistance. Sometimes respondents learned life skills or new perceptions that they found to be effective, but mostly, it was the characteristics of the relationships themselves which provided study participants the necessary impetus and capabilities to change their lives. The men's stories of desistance are presented in Chap. 2.

How specifically did these relationships function to assist respondents in changing their lives? Which mechanisms were at work and in which ways? What happened over time to create these changes?

Study data provided important information about the capabilities necessary for successful desistance to occur: an identity change, the construction of a life story in which the respondent evolved from a criminal to a prosocial community member, and relationships with prosocial others which provided critical affective and cognitive qualities. Respondents' desistance processes are detailed in Chap. 4.

Study results analyzing the mechanisms of significant relationships effective in facilitating desistance satisfied the dissertation requirements. However, there was much more to be learned from the men's narratives. Because their successful desistance processes were so much a product of their treatment experiences, the data could function as a guide in clinical work with these client populations. Hence, analysis of the data was incorporated into this book to develop a practice theory and treatment model for substance abusers and offenders based on the aspects of significant relationships that respondents found effective in helping them to attain desistance from criminal behavior and substance abuse.

Issues in Analyzing and Presenting the Data

One of the major obstacles to utilizing the self-report of offenders and substance abusers as qualitative data and a reliable source to generate conclusions is the respondents' propensity for deceitfulness. As a result of this concern, many researchers recommend obtaining confirmation from additional sources as a comparison and validation of self-report data (e.g., Elffers, 2010; Lindegaard,

2010). However, the Institutional Review Board which authorized this study did not permit employing any other source material such as criminal records or treatment documentation. Because the study's focus was on an internal psychological process, it was determined that self-report alone would provide sufficient information. Some researchers concur. In discussing interview-based research with offenders, Brookman (2010) asserted, "The further one moves from observable, factual events towards internal thoughts and perceptions, the less feasible and desirable validation becomes" (p. 95). Therefore, Curtis (2010) stated that it is possible to collect reliable self-report information from respondents who have engaged in stigmatizing or marginalizing behavior and that "more often than not they tell the truth" (p. 152). He said that researchers often get far more cooperation than they expect.

Results of qualitative studies such as this are not designed to be generalized or definitive. Although the desistance processes that study respondents described are utilized in this book to formulate a treatment model, it is not my intention to posit that all substance abusers and offenders will desist if these methods are employed. Substance abuse and criminal behavior can become areas of difficulty for many different reasons and for many different types of clients, and as such, their treatment needs will vary. The populations of those desisting from crime and substance abuse do not all respond to the same types of interventions, nor would they necessarily rely on interpersonal relationships in ways similar to this respondent group.

Generalizing or universalizing data is the task of quantitative methodology, research based on statistical analyses. Given the heterogeneity of the offender and substance abuser populations, I believe that evidence-based treatment derived from quantitatively based outcome studies can inadvertently lead to a "one size fits all" mentality of treatment intervention. Given the severity of substance abusers' and offenders' multiple psychological, behavioral, social, and cultural problems and stressors, one size does not fit all.

Psychodynamic Theory as a Framework to Explore Relational Dynamics

To formulate the practice model for this work, study results were integrated with a psychological theory to provide a framework for explaining and understanding the requisite individual and interpersonal processes leading to desistance. The practice model's functions are to apply the theoretical framework to the therapy process and explain how to develop treatment goals. Case examples presented based on the practice theory are drawn from study respondents' reports as well as descriptions from my clinical work. In order to remain consistent with the study's concentration on the mechanisms of interpersonal relationships in facilitating change, the theory chosen for this theoretical framework had to posit that the therapeutic relationship is the primary factor in psychic change.

Of the available psychologies of the mind, there is only one set of theories that focus clinical attention on the nature of the therapy relationship itself: those operating from a psychodynamic perspective. (For the purposes of this book, the terms psychoanalytic and psychodynamic are used interchangeably.) A central tenet connecting all psychodynamic theories is the assertion that the nature of the client-therapist relationship and the dynamic process between both parties is the main source of psychological and behavioral change (Bass, 2003; Benjamin, 2010; Holmes, 2011).

Psychodynamic theories share additional common ground that applies to the task of developing this practice theory. They maintain a focus on the internal psychological world, personality structure, and unconscious mental processes. They all "insist on the centrality of meaning-making" (Harris, 2010, p. 703). Clients must make sense of themselves and their worlds in order to change their thoughts, feelings, and behavior in a way that feels internally motivated and integrated with who they perceive themselves to be (Rothschild & Gellman, 2009). Gadd and Farrall (2004) stated that cognitive theory is not adequate to explain or understand offender desistance narratives; psychoanalytic theory must be employed to explain the role of unconscious motivation.

A recent addition to the psychoanalytic family, relational analytic theory was chosen as the theoretical framework for this project. Not a standalone theory, it is based on traditional object relations, ego psychology, intersubjectivity, attachment theory, and self psychology principles. An explanation of the tenets, concepts, and terminology applicable to all psychodynamic theory is outside the scope of this work. Those specific to the relational model are summarized in this chapter and more fully presented and explained in Chap. 3.

Although principles of the foundational theories, attachment, object relations, intersubjectivity, and self psychology, reflect the importance of relationships in personality development and overall mental health, they do so from a one-person standpoint with each individual contributing and gaining from the relationship. Relational analytic theory views human development as a co-created structure, asserting that early relationships with parents and caregivers are the primary organizer of character. Personality structure is viewed as emanating solely from identifications with attachment figures. Overwhelming aspects of these attachments cause dissociation and the development of fragmented self-states which undercuts their conscious accessibility. Here, individuals do not exist in isolation. In Winnicottian terms, there is no baby without the mother.

Accordingly, relational analytic theory views the therapeutic encounter as co-created between therapist and client. This theory asserts that the therapeutic relationship is the primary mechanism of change, situating "relations with others at the center of psychic life and places the patient-therapist relationship at the center of treatment" (Safran & Kraus, 2014, p. 386). Other psychodynamic theories portray the client as an individual with his or her issues and relational patterns, separate from the therapist's individuality. In this theory, the two are intertwined as a two-person entity. Client pathology is viewed as co-created by the therapeutic relationship. This stance changes the manner in which diagnostic assessments and treatment goals are formulated and significantly broadens possibilities for interventions which can be far more widely construed than interpretation alone.

Relational analytic theory's formulation of mental organization is particularly applicable to the psychological and interpersonal processes described by study respondents. This system of dissociation and fragmentation can easily account for conflicted motivation and the unconscious components of addiction and criminal behavior. It also provides a framework helpful in explaining the identity change process that offenders and substance abusers must experience in order to desist. The application of this theory to the development of respondents' criminal identities and substance abuse is explored in Chap. 3.

Strange Bedfellows

In the current treatment climate, offending, substance abuse, and psychoanalytic theory make strange bedfellows. The prevailing treatment of choice for those both with substance abuse problems and who commit crime is cognitive behavioral therapy (CBT). From this perspective, behaviors are viewed as emanating from dysfunctional thinking patterns. Most CBT-based treatment is comprised of a combination of psychoeducation, skills teaching, and limit setting with threats of discharge if attendance and treatment goals are not met. The sole focus is on behavioral change pertaining to the problem behavior. Treatment is often provided on a short-term basis and within a group modality (Ganzer & Ornstein, 2008).

Practitioners of CBT tend to view psychoanalytic theory as an anachronism. The "longstanding and sometimes antagonistic rift" between the substance abuse treatment community and psychodynamic practitioners (Rothschild & Gellman, 2009, p.28) also exists with those who espouse CBT treatment for criminals. The belief is that analytic therapy of offenders and substance abusers performed in the past produced little or no favorable results (Andrews & Bonta, 2010; Rothschild, 2010).

Perhaps this assertion is true. In its heyday during the mid-twentieth century, the goal of traditional psychoanalysis was insight. Following Freudian principles, pathological psychic defenses, the source of problem symptoms and behavior, existed to protect the person from overwhelming and unconscious drives. Once insight was attained, it was believed that the need for those defenses would dissipate along with their associated problematic symptomatology. The actual efficacy of analytic therapy provided for substance abusers and offenders during that time period is unknown.

Because its emphasis is on internal experience rather than external matters, psychodynamic therapy is notoriously difficult to evaluate (Miller, Luborsky, Barber, & Docherty, 1993). Concepts related to unconscious processing are not observable, nor are they easily measurable. Historically, the field has relied on case material as the main means of testing analytic hypotheses (Masling & Bornstein, 1994). At the time, evidence-based treatment as a facet of care did not exist. Furthermore, while the past prevalence of formal psychoanalysis for offenders and substance abusers has not been researched, it is informally acknowledged that analytic practitioners avoided clients with severe behavioral problems. They were not considered suitable subjects for analysis (Rothschild, 2010); neither were the poor (Gaztambide, 2012).

However, psychoanalytic theory has evolved since the mid-twentieth century, and the theories which emanated from Freud's original doctrine, object relations theory, ego psychology, attachment theory, self psychology, and relational analytic theory, include revisions to strict Freudian theory and therapy protocols. Interpretation, defined as those rare pronouncements from the supposedly neutral analyst which produce patient insight, has lost its grandiose status. With the advent of psychodynamically informed therapy, patients transformed into clients who did not lie down on couches or engage in freely associated discourses for 3–5 appointment hours per week. They sat up, physically, verbally, and symbolically. The concept of insight changed. It evolved to become a product of the therapeutic relationship, produced by the client as guided by the therapist, and focused on problem areas in the client's life.

Meanwhile, evidence-based protocols have been developed which permit evaluation of treatment outcomes for CBT-based treatment. While researchers, theorists, and practitioners argue among themselves about which set of treatment hypotheses and principles are most effective for these offender and substance abuser client populations, studies evaluating outcomes have reported equivocal results while rates of treatment success have remained stagnant (Dumaine, 2003; Fletcher, Nutton & Brend, 2015; Hubbard, Craddock, & Anderson, 2003; Wilson, 2014; Windsor, Jemal, & Alessi, 2015). It is time to revisit psychodynamic concepts as applicable to the treatment of offenders and substance abusers.

Treatment Models Which Integrate CBT and Psychodynamics

Recently, there have been attempts to integrate CBT's focus on thoughts and behaviors with aspects of treatment and personality traditionally considered to be within the realm of psychodynamic therapy. Some theorists and practitioners are considering attachment theory, the most popular (and evidence-based) of the psychodynamic theories, for use in treatment of substance abuse. For offenders and incarcerated populations, the risk-need-responsivity (RNR) model includes in its structure specifics regarding the quality of the therapeutic relationship which is viewed as an important mechanism of change. Both of these treatment models attend to the quality of the therapeutic relationship, requiring that the therapist establish a secure, caring, warm, and respectful stance with his or her clients.

Attachment theory focuses on personality traits that are developed based on the nature of the attachment between caregivers and young children. Its precepts have been tested empirically and found to be an accurate predictor of later adult pathology. Attachment theory was developed by John Bowlby (1982). Mary Ainsworth developed the research protocol for evaluating the veracity of attachment theory. For a summary of their collaborative work, see Ainsworth and Bowlby (1991). (Of course, rifts occur within fields as well as between them. Attachment theory was not considered to be a bona fide psychoanalytic theory until the past 20 years. See Fonagy (2001) for a comprehensive discussion of the history and attempts at integration of the two.)

Practitioners employing attachment theory in their work with substance abusers propose that substance abusers' early insecure attachments with significant others and the resulting characterological deficits are factors leading to reliance on substances. Drug and alcohol use is seen as a coping strategy used to anesthetize the pain from these inner wounds (Fletcher et al., 2015; Flores, 2004). This framework underscores the importance of constructing the therapeutic relationship as a secure attachment for clients. Furthermore, its precepts can be explained to clients as a cognitive framework to help them understand their present dysfunctional patterns in interpersonal relationships as well as their motivation to use substances. Coping strategies and other cognitive and behavioral methods can be employed within an attachment-based treatment model to help clients heal from their early dysfunctional relationships, achieve secure attachments in their present relationships, and consequently reduce the need for substance use.

The RNR model of treatment for offenders (Andrews & Bonta, 2010; Andrews, Bonta, & Wormith, 2011; Bonta & Andrews, 2007) incorporates three principles. Treatment intensity is based on the risk level of the client for reoffense. Criminogenic needs are targeted for treatment. Responsivity demands that programs be sensitive to the individual characteristics of their clientele such as their culture, motivation, and learning style (Olver, Wong, & Nicholaichuk, 2009). The principle of responsivity incorporates attention to issues of difference, such as race, ethnicity, socioeconomic status (SES), and sexual orientation. It includes as one of its precepts the necessity of developing and maintaining a warm, respectful, and collaborative working relationship with the client.

Empirical research on outcomes of the RNR model indicates that it is more effective than traditional CBT in treatment programs for incarcerated sex offenders. Hanson, Bourgon, Helmus, and Hodgson (2009) performed a meta-analysis of 23 recidivism outcome studies of sex offender programs that incorporated RNR principles into their treatment. They found these programs showed the largest reductions in sexual and general criminal recidivism, concluding that RNR principles should be a major consideration in the design and implementation of treatment programs for sex offenders.

A Relational Analytic Practice Model for Desisters

Given the mind's complexity, it seems illogical to compartmentalize thoughts, feelings, behaviors, relational needs, and conscious and unconscious motivation as separate mental functions and then determine that only some of these areas deserve theoretical and clinical attention. An effective practice protocol needs to address all aspects of the mind and behavior.

The application of relational analytic theory to therapeutic practice with substance abusers and offenders is discussed in Part III of the book. Chapter 5 explores the murky diagnostic issues relevant to these populations. The process of diagnosing is important as treatment is begun with this assessment. Due to limitations of the current diagnostic manuals, criteria and symptoms of the offending and substance abuse diagnoses are primarily behavioral in nature. They do not assist practitioners in formulating a comprehensive treatment plan.

Chapter 6 presents the practice theory and treatment model and the distillation of the theoretical framework into a usable form for therapy with these populations. Within it, care is taken to address the social and cultural issues relevant to these groups. The relationally based practice theory proposed in this book is designed as an organizing principle for therapists. It does not attempt to dictate what is said by either party; instead, it provides a context within which to understand what is said. Furthermore, it provides guidance about how to navigate the stormy interactional patterns, ebbs and flows of crises and demands, and sticking points that are hallmarks of treatment with these populations.

From the relational analytic perspective, the two most important functions within the therapy relationship are the processes of enactment and witnessing. Enactments, or crises, are understood as bringing forth into consciousness dissociated self-states representing the client's inner life and his or her painful experiences in close relationships. These relational patterns are brought to bear on the therapy relationship, activating the therapist's relational patterns. Enactments occur when both of these sets of relational patterns cause unconscious distress within the dyad, resulting in the disruption of the therapeutic holding environment. Interpersonal conflict between therapist and client ensues. The benefits of this seemingly negative occurrence are explained in Chap. 6.

Witnessing is a method of listening to clients. It is designed to address dissociation and personality fragmentation. Reparation of enactments and the process of witnessing provide the means to promote personal agency, the ability to set and achieve personal and behavioral goals. This treatment model is relationally based but it does not purport to be all things to all people. It can be utilized in parallel with existing CBT treatment protocols except for manualized treatment which predetermines the interaction between therapist and client.

Chapter 6 utilizes case examples to illustrate how relational principles work. Some clients have given me permission to use excerpts from their treatment in publications and presentations. I have also used clinical material from clients from whom I did not seek permission. In all cases, identifying information is masked. My goal was for any client reading this text to be unable to recognize himself if an example from his treatment were included.

Lastly, Chap. 7 applies this model to "real world" treatment situations and environments including short-term and group work taking place within publicly funded agencies and with mandated clients. Methods of integrating this relational framework with existing agency-based treatment programs are suggested.

References

Ainsworth, M. D. S., & Bowlby, J. (1991). An ethological approach to personality development. *American Psychologist, 46*, 333–341.

Andrews, D. A., & Bonta, J. (2010). *The psychology of criminal conduct* (5th ed.). Newark, NJ: Matthew Bender.

Andrews, D. A., Bonta, J., & Wormith, S. J. (2011). The risk-need-responsivity (RNR) model: Does adding the good lives model contribute to effective crime prevention? Criminal Justice and Behavior, 38, 735–755.

Bass, A. (2003). "E" Enactments in psychoanalysis: Another medium, another message. *Psychoanalytic Dialogues, 13*, 657–675.

Benjamin, J. (2010). Where's the gap and what's the difference? The relational view of intersubjectivity, multiple selves, and enactments. *Contemporary Psychoanalysis, 46*, 112–119.

Bonta, J., & Andrews, D. A. (2007). Risk-need-responsivity model for offender assessment and rehabilitation. *Rehabilitation, 6*, 1–22. Retrieved March 14, 2009, from http://www.publicsafety.gc.ca/res/cor/rep/risk_need_200706-eng.aspx.

Bowlby, J. (1982). *Attachment* (2nd ed.). New York: Basic Books. (Original work published 1969).

Brookman, F. (2010). Beyond the interview: Complementing and validating accounts of incarcerated violent offenders. In W. Bernasco (Ed.), *Offenders on offending: Learning about crime from criminals* (pp. 84–108). Devon, UK: Willan Publishing.

Curtis, R. (2010). Getting good data from people who do bad things: Effective methods and techniques for conducting research with hard-to-reach and hidden populations. In W. Bernasco (Ed.), *Offenders on offending: Learning about crime from criminals* (pp. 141–160). Devon, UK: Willan Publishing.

Dumaine, M. L. (2003). Meta-analysis of interventions with co-occurring disorders of severe mental illness and substance: Implications for social work practice. *Research on Social Work Practice, 13*, 142–165.

Elffers, H. (2010). Misinformation, misunderstanding, and misleading as validity threats to offenders' accounts of offending. In W. Bernasco (Ed.), *Offenders on offending: Learning about crime from criminals* (pp. 13–22). Devon, UK: Willan Publishing.

Fletcher, K., Nutton, J., & Brend, D. (2015). Attachment, a matter of substance: The potential of attachment theory in the treatment of addictions. *Clinical Social Work Journal, 43*, 109–117.

Flores, P. J. (2004). *Addiction as an attachment disorder*. Lanham, MD: Jason Aronson.

Fonagy, P. (2001). *Attachment theory and psychoanalysis*. New York: Other Press.

Gadd, D., & Farrall, S. (2004). Criminal careers, desistance and subjectivity: Interpreting men's narratives of change. *Theoretical Criminology, 8*, 123–156.

Ganzer, C., & Ornstein, E. D. (2008). In and out of enactments: A relational perspective on the short- and long-term treatment of substance abuse. *Clinical Social Work Journal, 36*, 155–164.

Gaztambide, D. J. (2012). Psychotherapy for the people. *Contemporary Psychoanalysis, 48*, 141–165.

Hanson, R. K., Bourgon, G., Helmus, L., & Hodgson, S. (2009). The principles of effective correctional treatment also apply to sexual offenders: A meta-analysis. *Criminal Justice and Behavior, 36*, 865–891.

Harris, A. E. (2010). The relational tradition: Landscape and canon. *Journal of the American Psychoanalytic Association, 59*, 701–735.

Holmes, J. (2011). Donnel Stern and relational psychoanalysis. *British Journal of Psychotherapy, 27*, 305–315.

Hubbard, R. L., Craddock, S. G., & Anderson, J. (2003). Overview of 5-year followup outcomes in the drug abuse treatment outcome studies (DATOS). *Journal of Substance Abuse Treatment, 25*, 125–134.

Lindegaard, M. R. (2010). Method, actor and context triangulations: Knowing what happened during criminal events and the motivations for getting involved. In W. Bernasco (Ed.), *Offenders on offending* (pp. 109–129). Collumpton, UK: Willan Publishing.

Masling, J. M., & Bornstein, R. F. (1994). *Empirical perspectives on object relations theory*. Washington, DC: American Psychological Association.

Miller, N. E., Luborsky, L., Barber, J. P., & Docherty, J. P. (1993). *Psychodynamic treatment research: A handbook for clinical practice*. New York: Basic Books.

Olver, M. E., Wong, S. C. P., & Nicholaichuk, T. (2009). Outcome evaluation of a high-intensity inpatient sex offender treatment program. *Journal of Interpersonal Violence, 24*, 522–536.

Rothschild, D. (2010). Partners in treatment: Relational psychoanalysis and harm reduction therapy. *Journal of Clinical Psychology: In Session, 66*, 136–149.

Rothschild, D., & Gellman, M. (2009). Finding the common ground: Contemporary psychoanalysis and substance abuse treatment. *Journal of Addictive Diseases, 28*, 28–38.

Safran, J. D., & Kraus, J. (2014). Alliance ruptures, impasses and enactments: A relational perspective. *Psychotherapy, 51*, 381–387.

Wilson, H. A. (2014). Can antisocial personality disorder be treated? A meta-analysis examining the effectiveness of treatment in reducing recidivism for individuals diagnosed with ASPD. *International Journal of Forensic Mental Health, 13*, 36–46.

Windsor, L. C., Jemal, A., & Alessi, E. J. (2015). Cognitive behavioral therapy: A meta-analysis of race and substance abuse outcomes. *Cultural Diversity and Ethnic Minority Psychology, 21*, 300–313.

2

The Men's Stories

Abstract Study respondents are introduced in this chapter. The research project's methodology and the 11 respondents' demographic information are summarized. The study sample included men living in the community for at least 3 years after an incarceration for violent behavior. Despite the commonalities of gender, criminal behavior, substance abuse, incarceration, and utilization of treatment, this group was diverse in terms of race, religion, years of incarceration, types of violent offenses, years in the community, education, and employment. The 11 sections of the chapter are devoted to each respondent's story. Information respondents shared about their families, early childhood, traumatic events, descent into crime, and encounters with the criminal justice system is presented. An overview of their turning points, beginning attempts at treatment, and desistance pathways is described.

Qualitative research methods where study participants are asked to share their personal experiences are best suited to explore an internal and interpersonal change process like desistance. The qualitative research interview supports respondents' change process because it is "a meaningful forum for identity expression" (Presser, 2008, p. 3). Additionally,

© The Editor(s) (if applicable) and The Author(s) 2016

D.H. Benveniste, *Changing Substance Abuse and Criminal Behavior Through Therapeutic Relationships*, DOI 10.1057/978-1-137-53039-4_2

the qualitative nature of this study gives voice to a marginalized group, one whose viewpoints and perspectives are rarely sought. Richardson (1990) describes narrative research of marginalized groups as "the textual enfranchisement of the previously disenfranchised" (p. 64). In spite of, or perhaps because of, the data being in the form of respondents' narrative self-report, qualitative data analysis follows a strict methodology.

Overview of Study Methodology

I first employed criminological and psychological theory to produce a framework from which my research question was developed: How do adult men who are desisting from committing acts of violence understand their desistance and the relationships that influence this process? A provisional code list based on previous studies comprising concepts referring to the impact of relationships on the desistance process was determined including: significant relationship; care, concern, and warmth; trust; guidance; support; sense of belonging; reframing negative self-states; and developing a prosocial identity.

The audio versions of the interviews were then transcribed into written transcripts. The transcripts were analyzed using qualitative data analysis software to search the written phrases and paragraphs for these provisional codes. Further codes were developed based on the narratives themselves. After the initial coding, I reviewed the transcripts again, revised the coding scheme, and reanalyzed the data. At this phase of the analysis, I looked for patterns of the desistance process, turning points into desistance, aspects of significant relationships that facilitated respondents' capacity to engage in these phases, and indicators of identity change. The final analysis integrated features of the literature, my practice experience, and the data. See the Appendix for further explanation of the study's methodology.

Beyond this methodological structure, the qualitative data analysis did not impose a theory onto what was shared. Data based on the men's narratives must be presented first in its true form before any further analysis can proceed. The application of relational theory to the interview data occurred after the fact and for the purposes of this book. Demographic information about the respondents is presented followed by their individual stories.

Demographic Information

The 11 men who consented to one-time interviews for this study were as similar as they were different. Each had been convicted of at least one act of violence and suffered societal ostracism pertaining to one or more cultural vulnerabilities including racial minority status, history of substance abuse and mental illness, being raised in poverty and urban ghettoes, and HIV disease. Within this common bond of societal marginalization, there were threads that connected most of the men. Ten had never been married, ten were heterosexual, and ten committed non-sexual offenses. Only one was homeless and one completed a college degree.

Beyond these basic commonalities however, much about the group was divergent. Criminal history, estimated length of time incarcerated, and years in the community since the last incarceration varied tremendously. Five respondents committed multiple, serious acts of violence; four committed one assault that did not involve the use of a weapon but was treated as serious by the criminal justice system; two committed multiple non-serious acts of violence. Non-serious violent acts are defined as brief interactions which do not inflict serious harm and do not involve the use of a weapon.

Five men spent less than 5 years incarcerated. Two of the respondents spent less than 1 year in prison while six spent over 6 years in prison. Three were imprisoned multiple times totaling more than 15 years of incarceration each. Four respondents had been living in the community for over 10 years at the time of the interview. Three had been released from prison less than 3 years before they met with me. Table 2.1 displays respondents' criminal histories.

Demographically, the men were diverse as well. Their ages ranged from 31 to 60, with six men between 41 and 50 years old. Eight were African American or a blend of African American and Caucasian or Native American. Three were Caucasian. Seven of 11 respondents were raised in urban ghettoes. Two grew up poor outside of major urban areas and two

Table 2.1 Respondents' reports of criminal histories, estimated length of time incarcerated, and years in the community since last incarceration

Variable	n (%)
Criminal history	
Long history, serious violence	5 (45%)
One violent crime	4 (36%)
Multiple non-serious violent acts[a]	2 (18%)
Domestic violence conviction	2 (18%)
Domestic violence report only	5 (45%)
Estimated length of time incarcerated	
Less than 1 year	2 (18%)
1–5 years	3 (27%)
6+ years	3 (27%)
Multiple incarcerations over 15+ years	3 (27%)
Years in the community since last incarceration	
3 years	3 (37%)
4–6 years	3 (27%)
7–9 years	1 (9%)
10+ years	4 (36%)

[a]A non-serious violent act is defined as a brief interaction which does not infl ct serious harm and does not involve the use of a weapon

were raised by middle-class families. Half the men reported no religion. Half reported no children. Half lived in their own apartments, three with intimate partners. Half of the respondents were high-school graduates. Half were unemployed or disabled and half worked full- or part-time. All but one of the respondents who were working full-time also volunteered. Most of those working part-time or who were unemployed volunteered. Although much of this unpaid work occurred as a product of 12 Step program involvement, respondents also served at local shelters and food kitchens. Table 2.2 displays demographic information.

Seven of 11 respondents received no mental health treatment. Three received both therapy and medication. Four men were HIV+. Table 2.3 displays information about respondents' health statuses.

Each man was asked to tell the story of his desistance from violence. Eleven unique stories emerged from this landscape. Narratives included respondents' background history, drug and alcohol usage, relationships with significant others, criminal and gang involvement, and court and incarceration experiences. Respondents described the turning points that

Table 2.2 Characteristics of the respondent group

Characteristic	n (%)
Age	
31–40	3 (27%)
41–50	6 (54%)
51–60	2 (18%)
Race	
African American	6 (54%)
Caucasian	3 (27%)
Blend	2 (18%)
Religion	
Christian	4 (36%)
Muslim	2 (18%)
None	5 (45%)
Number of children	
0	5 (45%)
1–2	4 (36%)
3+	2 (18%)
Marital status	
Never married	7 (63%)
Married	1 (9%)
Cohabitating	3 (27%)
Sexual orientation	
Heterosexual	10 (90%)
Homosexual	1 (10%)
Educational status	
High school not completed	2 (18%)
High school graduate	6 (54%)
Some college	2 (18%)
Associate degree	1 (9%)
Employment status	
Part-time	3 (27%)
Full-time	3 (27%)
Unemployed	3 (27%)
Disabled	2 (18%)
Childhood living situation	
Inner city	7 (63%)
Poor	2 (18%)
Middle class	2 (18%)

Table 2.3 Health status: substance abuse, mental illness, and HIV disease

Variable	n (%)
Type of substance abuse	
None	1 (9%)
Alcohol and marijuana	1 (9%)
Polysubstance abuse	9 (81%)
Substance abuse treatment	
Detox	9 (81%)
AA or NA	7 (63%)
Sober house	4 (36%)
Halfway house	2 (18%)
Counseling while incarcerated	1 (9%)
Outpatient counseling	1 (9%)
Mental health treatment	
Therapy and medication	3 (27%)
Therapy only	1 (9%)
None	7 (63%)
HIV status	
Positive	4 (36%)
Negative	7 (63%)

forced them to observe and assess the course of their lives. They discussed their efforts to learn and integrate new methods of coping and behavior which support a sober and crime-free lifestyle and the relationships which facilitated this change. The men are referred to by their nicknames, chosen by them before the interview process began.

Narratives

The Only Thing You Have to Change Is Everything

Jay was 46 years old at the time of his interview, having spent most of his adult life in and out of prison. He is African American and Native American and comes from an intact family with five siblings: two sisters and three brothers. As an early teen, Jay became involved with gangs, explaining this behavior as modeling his father and brothers. He used alcohol and marijuana but it was when he was incarcerated at age 18 that he discovered heroin. Over the next two decades, Jay said he did not see a way out of this life. It was "us against the world" and "everyone on the other side was assholes." At first, he avoided any form of treatment. He did not trust others and was suspicious of anyone who attempted to intervene. However, as his sentences became longer, Jay would attend treatment programs as a means to avoid further incarceration.

Jay's turning point occurred over time and involved several factors. The first was a critical interaction with one of his brothers. One day as Jay sat in a court lockup awaiting sentencing, he saw his brother, also in lockup awaiting sentencing, who announced that he was done with criminal activity. Since Jay had often heard this proclamation from others facing prison, he did not pay it much mind. However, his brother did not return to his previous lifestyle after that. As Jay watched his other brothers and father leave behind a criminal lifestyle, he began to be charged as a persistent felony offender, an offense imposing a mandatory sentence of 60 years. Additionally, he was diagnosed HIV+ at age 43. As Jay was contemplating a change in his life course, he began a treatment program which he described as having a major impact on his thinking.

> They made you do a whole family tree, so you went through everyone in your family, from your grandmothers, your father's side, mother's side, everyone. Then you sat up in front of a group and you went through that whole process, your relationships with all of them. Then it was a criminal history thing you went through, and the addiction. And when I was doing that addiction, the director came in there. And she took my file and she sat there. And she stopped the group, and she's like, 'Well I'm gonna tell you, I know a lot of people is not going to agree, but you just got to stop going to jail.'
>
> And that's something I never heard. It was always drugs was the problem. So I'm like, 'What do you mean?' She was like, 'You've been in jail more than you have been addicted to drugs, in your active addiction.' And I'm looking at it, and it's clear to me. My time in jail was outweighing my—you know and it's like wow. She was like, 'You know, you got to really concentrate on that, you know and what's making you do those behaviors'. That's basically my thinking, thinking I can get away with this or that or to get something for nothing, you know, all of that. It's just tied in.

From there, he applied for and was accepted into a residential program for those who are HIV+.

He began to work the Narcotics Anonymous (NA) program including sharing his fears and "what was really going on with him." He reported that he was speaking to his sponsor and his brother every day and working as an aide in a homeless shelter in addition to volunteer jobs in a soup kitchen and grassroots substance abuse agency. About the nature of the change process, Jay stated:

> I was willing to go all out. I remember the guy actually being my sponsor, he said,
>
> 'The only thing you have to change is everything.' That didn't sit well with me, you know, change everything. I know I've got some good things. I didn't understand what he was saying. Now I do, you know.

At the time of the interview, Jay reported having been crime- and drug-free for 3 years, after successfully completing parole for the first time in his life.

She Sees

Pink Panther (a nickname based on his favorite cartoon character) was 57 years old at the time of the interview and unemployed. He is African-American and was raised in the inner city by an intact family. The youngest of four children, he said that the other three were doing well. Pink Panther explained that when he was a youngster, his mother would tell him stories of his father being an alcoholic and beating her. However, he stated that he did not witness this behavior as it had stopped by the time he was born. Pink Panther started using hard liquor and marijuana at age 14 and experimented with pills during his teens. He said "then crack cocaine came along and ruined my life." He said he was using as well as dealing the drug. He moved down south where his family is from to escape the triggers that surrounded him but found himself engaged in the same behaviors there.

Mid-way through the interview, Pink Panther said that he could not focus on what I was asking because he had too much on his mind. I asked what he would like to talk about and he said he needed to talk about his girlfriend who had died in his arms 3 years before. He went on to relate that she suffered from congestive heart failure secondary to extensive drug abuse and HIV illness. He said that they had lived together for 14 years, she on disability and he working part time but both using crack cocaine together. He said she would "flip out" because she would want more drugs and would "put her hands on him" out of frustration. He would retaliate and grab her.

Pink Panther recalled that during one fight in 2008, he grabbed her so hard that he bruised her. She called the police and obtained a restraining order. Pink Panther was arrested for hitting his girlfriend and served a 90-day sentence. He said he would have had to serve only 45 days but he had written a letter of apology to her while incarcerated. After she brought it to her case manager, he was sentenced to another 45 days for violating the restraining order. She took him back after he was released and died shortly thereafter.

Pink Panther's turning point occurred as a result of the loss of his girlfriend. After her death, he found himself homeless. His girlfriend's daughter, his sister, and his brother all offered him a place to stay but for the first time in his life, he said he wanted his own place and to be "independent." At the same time, he began to attempt treatment. He went to detox twice but when faced with the need for treatment a third time, he decided "three strikes and you're out" and detoxed himself.

Pink Panther returned to Alcoholics Anonymous (AA) but used the program differently than in the past, this time "getting the commitment" and sharing about himself. He also applied for mental health treatment, saying, "I have major depression in my life." He described his psychiatrist and therapist as very helpful to him. He was in the application processes for Social Security Disability and housing. Pink Panther reported being prescribed psychotropic medication but not taking it regularly because he said that it slowed him down too much. However, he did say that it helped stabilize his mood, keeping him "balanced." He was volunteering regularly and stayed "humble" saying that he appreciated what others did for him. One of the major motivators he described for his current sobriety and crime-free lifestyle was his girlfriend saying, "the longer I stay clean, the happier she will be because she sees." At the time of the interview, Pink Panther reported being violence-free for 4 years and sober for 5 months.

You Ain't That Dude No More

Black is not the kind of man to sit and talk about himself or his life. He said, "I'm not really a verbal type of guy. This is the most you'll hear me talk probably ever." He described a difficult childhood in the projects of a major urban area. He is African-American and was raised by his mother and "step pops" who were both alcoholic and spent their weekends partying and fighting. He said that his mother spent her adolescence in a facility for juvenile delinquents. He did not discuss his biological father. Black had two brothers, one who was given up for adoption as a baby and one who is a year older than Black. He said that when he was age 17, his older brother returned to the family at age 19 but was killed by his girlfriend 5 years later at age 24. As a result of his upbringing and experiences, Black determined early on that "instead of being the victim, be the victimizer. So instead of being hurt, I'd rather hurt first."

Black said he was violent with his girlfriends because he saw others treat women in that way. He began to steal, rob, and use and sell drugs as a teenager and was first incarcerated at age 16. Black was 43 years old at the time of the interview and had spent a total of 18 years incarcerated. He described that he would get out of prison, try to remain crime-free but return to using and dealing drugs within a couple of months. He was embarrassed to admit that he was quite comfortable in prison.

Black's turning point occurred 4 years prior to the interview when he discovered that his mother was terminally ill. With 18 days left to his sentence, he was offered a choice: either to be escorted to the hospital to see her or be brought to her funeral. He opted for the hospital visit and was shocked to see her condition. His family had chosen not to disclose the extent of her illness to him because he was incarcerated. He recalled being very angry at first but said he realized that he was not "an innocent bystander," believing that the stress induced by his lifestyle was a factor in causing her cancer. He described that his mother had always taken care of him when he was incarcerated by sending him money and taking his phone calls. Once she died, he said to himself, "I definitely got to do something different!"

Shortly thereafter, Black married his long-term girlfriend and they had a son. Black described working hard to change his thinking. He said he had to learn to let his wife guide his behavior and actively talk himself out of going for fast money because of the consequences.

Black could not find work due to his criminal history and lack of work experience. He said that this situation caused him considerable frustration particularly as his wife sometimes worked two jobs. However, as a result, Black found himself taking care of their son. At the time of the interview, Black had been his son's primary caregiver for 4 years, a source of pride and responsibility. He said that when his wife asks their son what color something is and he answers correctly, Black thinks to himself. "Yeah, that's *my* work."

Recently, Black found himself in his hometown and his old neighborhood. As he watched the goings on, he thought to himself, "You ain't that dude no more." At the time of the interview, Black had been crime-free and sober for 4 years.

I Didn't Know Who to Trust

Dee was one of the younger respondents, 33 years old at the time of the interview. He reported that he came from a "good" family; his parents were together and he has three brothers, two older and one younger. He described being raised in a middle-class family in a small city. Dee's father is African-American and his mother is Caucasian. He initially described his family as healthy, without any abuse, but later reported that one of his older brothers bullied him when he was young, an experience to which he ascribed his lifelong anger. Dee also reported that he is gay and was insecure about his sexuality. He said that he had attended some college and worked consistently in restaurant management.

Dee's drug abuse and violent behavior first began during his twenties and he believed that it was relationship-based; he was either getting into violent altercations with his partners or with the partners of his female friends when he was asked to intervene. Shortly after his first arrest, he discovered that his partner was HIV+ and had given Dee the AIDS virus. Dee described his response as being "Angry at the world and angry at myself" After multiple probation sentences, he was incarcerated once for a year and began using marijuana after his release. He described becoming involved with another man who was not "out" and that they used cocaine, angel dust, and heroin together. Dee recalled that he desperately needed to talk to someone about his anger and HIV status but did not know whom to trust.

Dee's turning point occurred after being hospitalized for HIV-related pneumonia. From there, he began drug treatment in a 28-day detox program. He moved out on his own and got another job but found himself in the same situation: using drugs, angry at the world, and unable to talk to anyone about his status. This time, rather than losing his temper, he quit the job before he began getting into altercations and applied for admission to a long-term sober house for people with HIV. He immediately requested and obtained a mental health therapist whom he described as helpful. He also talked about feeling acceptance and self-esteem for the first time because everyone in the sober house was HIV+. Dee reported that he was planning to return to school to be a substance abuse and HIV counselor. At the time of the interview, he had been violence-free for 5 years, sober for more than a year, and had successfully completed probation 3 months before.

The Right Frame of Mind

Ace was age 57 at the time of the interview and African-American. He said he was one of eight children but the "black sheep" as all of his siblings were doing well, some of whom he was proud to say were artists. He said when he was young, he watched his cousins "be hustlers and players and stuff" and that several of them were pimps. He said he was "always in trouble as a kid," stealing cars, breaking into people's houses, and committing robberies.

Ace said he found women fascinating and "wanted to be around them." He used prostitutes often and sometimes would not pay them. He reported that one prostitute filed assault charges against him and although he vehemently denied accosting her, he said the police found a carpet knife among the carpet-installing tools in his trunk (from his employment) and arrested him. Ace said he was offered a plea bargain of 8 years with four to serve but he chose to go to trial, believing that he would be acquitted because he was not guilty. Instead, he was given the entire original 12-year sentence of which he served 6 years. This was his last violent offense.

After his incarceration, Ace reported that he met a woman who was a drug addict and became involved with her. He said he became addicted to crack cocaine at that time because he "had to do it or leave her and I needed somebody to hang onto." Ace struggled with addictions to alcohol, marijuana, and cocaine over the next several years.

At 5 or 6 AM one morning, Ace found himself aimlessly walking down the street. He had been using crack cocaine and had lost both his job and his car as a result. He said that his niece saw him while on her way to work. She called her mother, his sister, who went to pick him up and told him "he was not leaving her sight" until she got him into treatment. He said she arranged admission to an inpatient program for him. Ace described his turning point as beginning at this juncture.

Ace went to the program but said he did not like it. During a stint in a sober house, he realized he had focused on the wrong aspect of the program and began reading the Bible. He became closer with his sister and started attending church where his niece was singing in the choir. One day after church, Ace, his sister, his niece, and his niece's friend went to breakfast and during the course of the meal, both his niece and her friend referred to him as "Uncle Ace." He said he was struck by the realization that they looked up to him and because they saw something good in him, he wanted to be a role model for them. Ace said he then realized that the most important part of his recovery was to volunteer and help others. He said if he is doing the right things and in the right frame of mind, he could encourage others to do the same.

Ace was working part-time as a landscaper at the time of the interview after having recently lost a good job with a college dining service when they discovered he was on the sex offender registry. At this time, he reported having been violence-free for 12 years and substance-free for nine.

One Handprint Closer to a Change of Heart

Brother Nowapo, age 48, began his narrative by stating that at the age of 12, he witnessed the murder of his father and that he never got any therapy to deal with that experience. He is African-American and went on to describe a traumatizing childhood in a very poor and violent section of a major urban area. In addition to his own father, Brother Nowapo reported that his half sister's father and Brother Nowapo's son were both killed as a result of this violence. He began his criminal career as an early teen serving as a lookout for a drug operation but recalled that he quickly moved to robbing the drug dealers themselves and using and selling cocaine and heroin.

At age 19, Brother Nowapo was sentenced to 55 years and served a total of 26 years. He continued to use and sell drugs and fight during the incarceration. He was sentenced to an additional year for stabbing another inmate. Upon release, he went to the doctor because he was "tired all the time" and found that he was HIV+. He reported that he assaulted both the doctor because he was angry about being HIV+ and the father of the woman he thought had given him the disease. However, he realized that he did not want to return to jail.

Brother Nowapo said his turning point occurred when he went to an AIDS task force where a case manager referred him to a sober house for people with HIV located in another state. He entered this program but left after an altercation with the program director. He did not do well on his own and soon requested readmission. He stated that the new program director was the most instrumental person in his recovery because she gave him a second chance and accepted him back. This time, he said he was working hard at self-care. He was attending AA regularly, taking HIV and psychotropic medication, and eating carefully as he reported he had also had two strokes. He was on Social Security Disability and volunteered at a soup kitchen.

Struggling with guilt about his previous behavior, Brother Nowapo described working hard to avoid responding aggressively when upset or frustrated. He talked about the importance of his mental health therapist, proudly stating that they had been meeting for 3 years. He said that he and his therapist set goals for him and that meeting those goals helped him to see himself as a better person and productive member of society. His plan was to go to school to become a substance abuse counselor.

Brother Nowapo also discussed the impact of his family and their religious beliefs on his desistance, describing them as very supportive and encouraging since he cleaned up. He shared a parable, One Handprint Closer to a Change of Heart, told to him by his brother and from which he was basing his new sense of self:

> This man who was a murderer had 99 murders and he wanted to change so he went to one man and said, "How can I change?" And the man said, "You can't change because you're a murderer" so he killed him, too. So he had a hundred murders. But he went to another wise old man and he said, "You have to move from this land and you have to have a change of heart and when you do that, you'll become a better person and you won't be a murderer anymore." As he traveled on his journey, he ended up in a desert where he left his handprint. The Angel of Death came down and said, "This is my soul" but the Great Architect of the Universe intervened and sent the Angel of Mercy who said, "This is my soul and I am going to measure where he was coming from to where he was going. He was one handprint closer to having a change of heart." So that's how he changed. And that's how I am. I want to be one handprint closer to having a change of heart.

After being incarcerated between the ages of 19 and 45, at the time of the interview, Brother Nowapo reported being violence-free for 3 years and crime-free and sober for two.

Comfort Zone

The youngest member of the respondent group at 31 and Caucasian, Nick (his clever response to the request for a nickname) was the only one without a substance abuse history. He said he had been on Social Security Disability for mental health since age 18. Nick reported that his mother suffered from major mental illness. He has two brothers, one of whom molested him when they were young. At age eight, Nick was removed from his mother's care by the state and was raised in psychiatric residential programs. He was released from the state's care at age 17 and after his release from the residential program, he returned home to live with his mother. Nick sadly reported that a couple of months later, he discovered her dead on the floor. He said he was evicted from the apartment by his older brother and moved in with a girlfriend where he lived for several years until the incident occurred which landed him in prison.

Nick described that he got into a fight with an older man who had punched his girlfriend in the jaw. He said he hit him three times and walked away. The assault on an elderly person carried a mandatory year sentence but he said the charge was reduced to a misdemeanor and he served 30 days. Nick reported that he was raped while in jail, an utterly traumatizing experience. His turning point resulted from the sexual abuse he experienced while incarcerated. He said after his release, he successfully completed 2 years of probation and never committed another criminal act in the ensuing 11 years.

Nick reported that at the time of the interview, he had been homeless for 2 years while awaiting subsidized housing. He opted not to sleep in shelters because he was afraid of the other people. He said he slept at friends' houses for a few days at a time, eating at a soup kitchen, and attending a psychiatric day program where he went as a child with his mother. He attributed his successful avoidance of aggressive behavior to "therapy, taking meds, learning techniques to deal with stress, and learning to walk away from situations that can get me into trouble." He said that he avoids the frustrated and angry people who populate the programs he attends and that over the years, he had learned to have patience with people.

However, Nick recalled an incident with his older brother that he could not avoid. His brother had wanted to drive with him out of town but Nick panicked and jumped out of the car because the town where he lived was his "comfort zone" and he was too afraid to leave. He said he saw his brother several days later who screamed at him for his impulsive behavior. Nick said he surprised himself by being able to calmly talk the situation through with his brother and repair the relationship. That was the first time he said he was able to cope with another's aggression in a healthy manner.

Set of Instructions

E was the most articulate of the group about his history and internal psychic processes, the result of a combination of innate intelligence, early psychiatric intervention, and multiple substance abuse treatment attempts. He described himself as a professional client. E is Caucasian,

36 at the time of the interview, and the youngest of three children, with two much older siblings close in age to each other. His mother had a major mental illness and was an alcoholic. He said that his maternal grandmother was a violent schizophrenic, in and out of psychiatric facilities, who eventually took her own life.

E's father left the family when E was 8 years old which precipitated his mother's decompensation. His older siblings had already left home by then. Left alone with his mother, she became physically abusive and neglectful toward him. E recalled that he was "fascinated with violence" from a young age, becoming "excited" watching fights. He described himself as the school bully in elementary school and that he "started getting diagnosed with things." The situation deteriorated until he was 12, when his mother broke his fingers slamming his hand into a car door. He was taken to the ER, removed from her care, and went to live with his father.

Although E was strongly attached to his father, he described him as a man who was not paying attention to his son. E began using and selling drugs in his teens. He said he was running a drug factory, growing marijuana out of his father's house, but that his father did not notice. As he was describing it to me, E remained unaware that this lack of oversight was neglectful on his father's part. By the time E was 17, he had a significant felony history and by the time he was 21, he had spent over 3 years in prison.

E's turning point occurred during the last of these incarcerations. He reported that his father came to see him and told him that he was not proud of him, that E was not the son he had raised, and that he was terminally ill with cancer. It was then that E decided to stop being violent and finished his sentence without incident. He said that although he never behaved violently again, he spent the next 6 years struggling with his drug and alcohol addictions. He chose to attend a treatment program rather than to return to prison for a probation violation and began a treatment merry-go-round, six programs in 4 months, using heroin and cocaine, getting a detox, getting out, using again, and returning to treatment until the last program "stuck."

E mentioned two factors that were instrumental in helping him to achieve and maintain sobriety: he now has a son who he actively parents and adores and AA and his sponsor provide him with the tools to maintain sobriety. For example, he said that his sponsor helped him to perceive his mother as doing the best she could, and as a result, his resentment toward her disappeared. About AA, he said:

> Most people don't have a plan or a solution or tools. They just sort of try and figure out life. I kind of feel privileged to be an alcoholic or an addict because I have a set of instructions that is in black and white and I haven't had anything happen in my life since I got sober that those instructions didn't handle.

E was hired as an assistant program coordinator for the program that provided his treatment and worked his way up, eventually becoming employed by the agency that funds the programs. At the time of the interview, E had been violence-free for 13 years and sober and working full-time for 5 years.

Growing Bonds

By the time Lee, who is African American, was 44, he had spent 25 years of his life drinking, using drugs, fighting, and going in and out of prison. He said he started drinking and using marijuana as a teen and dropped out of high school because he was "always partying." He started using cocaine when he was 20 and was addicted by the time he was 22. Lee said that when in "his right mind" he is not violent but under the influence, he has a short fuse. He said that his last incarceration was for 3 years for assaulting a police officer and that he was released from prison 3 years before this interview.

Lee described his years of sobriety prior to this incarceration. He was living in a sober house for HIV+ residents for 3 years and then on his own for 1 year, sober and working four part-time jobs. Lee said that he knows what to do to stay clean: attend AA meetings, keep AA commitments, and talk regularly to a sponsor, but that he has an additional addiction which interferes with his sobriety. He said he always longs for a romantic relationship, saying he needs to "feel that love" and becomes so "fascinated" that it "causes his downfall." He described that he would meet a woman who was in early recovery, become involved with her, change his focus from his own sobriety to hers, and end up drinking. He said that as a result of these episodes,

99% of the time, he would end up back in jail. He ascribed his addiction to relationships as the cause of his last failure to maintain sobriety.

Lee's turning point has been a slowly building affair, culminating in an unusual interaction with the criminal justice system. He requested and was granted readmission to the sober house where he had done so well previously and was able to transfer there directly after this most recent sentence was completed. Although he continued to drink and was arrested for public drunkenness, he did not engage in any further violent behavior. He said he had amassed three drinking in public charges that occurred close in time and decided to leave the sober house to go to detox, where he spent 45 days. After he completed the program, he went to court and faced the charges. The prosecutor informed the judge that Lee had not been before them in 2 years when it had previously been commonplace for them to see him in court four to five times per year. The judge had a letter from the detox facility indicating that Lee had done well in the program, and to Lee's amazement, he dismissed all the charges.

After this encouragement from the court, Lee reconciled with both his mother and his son who had "wanted nothing to do with him" when he was drinking. His son also had not permitted Lee to see his three young grandchildren. Lee described his guilt at not being there for his son when he was young and blamed himself for his son's drug problems as a teen. Lee said he would cry at AA meetings about this situation. He said the emotional pain would cause urges to drink but he realized doing so would keep his family from him longer. Now that they were reconciled, he adamantly stated that he would not do to his grandchildren what he did to his son. He said, "I'm growing a bond with them but at the same time I'm growing a bond with him, too." Furthermore, he also said that he was avoiding intimate relationships until he "feels secure within himself." At the time of the interview, Lee reported having been violence-free for 3 years and sober for 4 months.

They Seen Something in Me

Bama, a nickname based on his thick Southern accent, is Caucasian and was 42 at the time of the interview. He did not discuss his early history or his family other than to say he was raised around alcohol. Bama began the interview by discussing two very bad decisions culminating in a 35-year prison sentence. He reported that he had gotten drunk while in jail, locked a guard in his cell, and escaped. He escaped again from the same jail several months later by digging a tunnel to the outside. Bama was charged with escape with force, escape, and being a habitual offender and was transferred to a maximum security facility.

Bama said he drank steadily for the first 6 years of this incarceration, making and selling the brew while inside. Then slowly, he began to realize the necessity of doing something different with his life. He got his GED, the General Equivalency Diploma, an exam-based substitute for a high school diploma, and a certificate in carpentry. He applied and was accepted to a faith-based honor dorm where he tutored other inmates. Eventually, Bama got the job as the warden's "runner" by working hard to establish the trust he had lost from his behavior in jail. The warden rewarded him by recommending that the parole board see him even though he was not eligible at the time. He was granted parole after serving 10 years.

Bama completed his parole and spent the next several years remaining attached to nothing but alcohol. He would hop trains, stop where he liked, work for a period of time, and then leave when the urge struck him. He said it was "not nothing for me to go the store and never come back." During this time, he was incarcerated for brief stints for public intoxication or hopping trains but not for violent behavior.

Bama's turning point occurred when he found out that his mother had moved to the Northeast and was sick. He arrived in her city of residence but could not find her. He moved to a small city where he had once lived and was offered a job where he had previously been employed. Bama was sober for several months during a stay at a sober house but once he moved out on his own, he began drinking. He said he thought about hopping trains again but decided instead to get a detox. He had met a woman, the first woman he had ever dated sober, who had offered him a choice to either return to his previous life or get sober again and be with her. Bama chose her and they moved in together. He said he was attending AA meetings regularly, telling his story, and doing commitments such as greeting people and bringing cookies. He also had a sponsor. At the time of the interview, Bama reported being violence-free for 10 years, crime-free and sober for 16 months, and had quit smoking cigarettes the month before we met.

From Birth to Death

Mark was both the most stable and accomplished of the respondent group. He was working full-time as a client supervisor for the private non-profit halfway house program he attended as part of his prison sentence. He had just celebrated his 10-year anniversary of employment there and Mark reported that he was crime- and substance-free during this period. He has an associate's degree and was living with a woman and raising their two children with her. Mark is African-American and aged 44 at the time of the interview. He was the only respondent who wanted me to use his real name and not a nickname. (I was unable to comply due to confidentiality rules of the study. 'Mark' is his nickname.)

Mark said that he, along with his one brother, was raised in "the projects" by a single mother. He reported that his mother beat both of them in an unsuccessful attempt to instill discipline. He did not know his father at all. He disclosed that when he was 7 or 8, he was molested by an older girl and that this experience terrified him.

Mark described himself as a product of his environment and reported that he was involved in a lot of non-violent criminal activity as a teen, primarily stealing. He said he would drink or smoke marijuana beforehand due to fear. He said he engaged in relationships with older women when he was a teen, one in which he was exposed to cocaine. Mark said he spent his twenties "drinkin', chasin' girls, and gettin' high." He had two children by two different women. At age 27, Mark was sentenced to 3 years for "kicking in his girlfriend's door and threatening to kill her with a knife." He served 2 years in prison and was transferred to a treatment-oriented halfway house for the last year.

Mark's turning point began prior to the arrest which led to this incarceration. He said he was thinking to himself that he was "tired of living like this" and it was "on his mind to try to change." His final decision occurred immediately after this arrest. He said he knew he was done. Mark said he experienced excruciating loneliness while imprisoned and decided he would never choose to live that way again.

With a wry and self-deprecating sense of humor, Mark described the impact of treatment in changing his thought processes and behavior.

He said he realized that in his past life, he was "an asshole." He said he "learned in a program that if your words and your action don't match, it's not really gonna work out." It was in treatment that he first disclosed his sexual victimization. He learned that using substances was an attempt to cope with overwhelming feelings and how his emotions connect to his behavior. He began to understand the profound effect on him of being raised without a father. Mark also had to learn to treat women differently. He said he learned that he had been "misinformed his whole life" about women and knew that he wanted a stable home and to raise children.

When he was released from his sentence, Mark committed himself to living a different lifestyle. He did not know how to go about it, so he reported that he relied on the judgment and guidance of his therapists. He said:

> I was willing to do anything on the other side. My mentality was, when I went to that program, it didn't matter what they told me to do to stay out, I was gonna do it. If they told me, 'You know what, Mark, stand on your head and spit nickels' then fine, that's what I'm doin'. 'Mark, you shouldn't go live over there.' 'Where should I live at?' 'Well there's a…' 'All right. Then I'm there.' I took whatever suggestions they offered cause I can't say I'm gonna do this and then act like that.

At the time of the interview, Mark was working three jobs: a full-time client supervisor position, and two part-time aide positions, one with the developmentally delayed and one in home health care. He was living with a woman with whom he had two children, a son age 6 and a daughter age 2. He was an active and emotionally engaged father. By then, he had three children from previous relationships. Mark talked about his commitment to raise his young children and his concomitant guilt about not having done so for his three older children. His oldest son was incarcerated at the time of the interview. About that, Mark said, "I taught him how to go to jail. I live with that guilt every day."

When tempted toward his old life, Mark reminds himself, "I have a family at home and I see how my son and my daughter are at home, especially my son. I think, if I take myself out of his life, this is gonna ruin him and I think, 'Damn, I wish I had somebody to do this for me when I was his age.' And I see that and I remember that was another one of my goals when I got out: that I was gonna have a child and raise him from birth to death." But Mark also knows that the old lifestyle is never far away. He said, "Damn, I still have a long way to go. You know what I mean? I don't do a lot of things but I haven't forgotten how to do what I used to do."

Summary

Several themes emerged from participants' stories, those which enabled crime and substance abuse as well as the path away from those behaviors and lifestyles. Many shared a traumatic and dysfunctional childhood; one marred by poverty, substance abuse, physical and sexual abuse, and death. Most became crime and substance-involved during the tumultuous developmental period of adolescence. Aggression toward intimate partners was learned from older relatives or peers. Numerous respondents were facing a life in prison. Chapter 3 begins the analysis of respondents' narratives using relational theory concepts and explores the role of dissociation in the development of their criminal identities.

References

Presser, L. (2008). *Been a heavy life: Stories of violent men*. Urbana: University of Illinois Press.

Richardson, L. (1990). Writing strategies: Reaching diverse audiences. In P. K. Manning, J. Van Maanen, & M. L. Miller (Eds.), *Qualitative research methods series* (Vol. 21). Newbury Park, CA: Sage Publications.

Part II

Relational Analytic Theory and Desistance

This section of the book is composed of three areas: the presentation of relational analytic theory, its application to study respondents' onset of criminal behavior and substance abuse, and an analysis of respondents' narratives exploring their desistance pathways. Chapter 3 discusses relational concepts basic to the desistance process and links this material to respondents' descriptions of their early life, exploring how trauma and dissociation produced aggressive and antisocial self-states. In Chap. 4, the author provides an analysis of study respondents' narratives to explore their desistance pathways. Emphasis is placed on the role of significant relationships in facilitating desistance from criminal behavior and substance abuse. The process of identity change is explored including its cognitive, affective, and behavioral components. Societal obstacles to desistance are discussed.

3

Theoretical Context

Abstract Relational theory derives from psychoanalytic theories including self-psychology, object relations, intersubjectivity, and attachment theory. It incorporates basic psychodynamic principles including internalization of objects, splitting, projective identification, and countertransference as non-verbal communication. What distinguishes relational theory from its predecessors is its view of mental organization. Departing from Freud's horizontal structures of id, ego, and superego, relational theory posits that dissociation creates vertical fissures in the mind producing disconnected self-states. Whole swaths of personality are disengaged from one's conscious sense of self leading to identity diffusion and psychopathology. Dissociation occurs in response to early childhood trauma and deficiencies in caretaking. Respondents' narratives are analyzed from this theoretical perspective. The author posits that criminal behavior and substance abuse are behaviors associated with particular dissociated self-states.

In order to explore the themes relevant to this study—life stories, the conception of identity, self-states, and the internal processes involved in identity and behavioral change—it is necessary to utilize a theoretical framework that addresses all of these complex concepts as well as an

© The Editor(s) (if applicable) and The Author(s) 2016

D.H. Benveniste, *Changing Substance Abuse and Criminal Behavior Through Therapeutic Relationships*, DOI 10.1057/978-1-137-53039-4_3

exploration of the dynamics of the therapy relationship and its change mechanisms. The first part of this chapter introduces the basic concepts of relational analytic theory relevant to the desistance process. The second part examines the relational themes present in study respondents' narratives and applies these principles to a developmental explanation of their ongoing struggles with criminal behavior and substance abuse.

Psychodynamic theory is the best choice for this exploration due to its emphasis on conscious and unconscious forces of attachment that form personality and produce change. Yet the psychoanalytic theories utilized during the early twentieth century such as drive theory, ego psychology, and object relations are insufficient for this endeavor as well. These theories sought only to explain the internal workings of the individual mind. Furthermore, although these theories were considered a radical concept at the time, they are now generally viewed as best suited for the worried (and wealthy) well. Many current analytical theorists and practitioners consider clients with multiple psychological, behavioral, social, and cultural stressors to be "unanalyzable" (Altman, 2005).

Relational Analytic Theory

A recent innovation in the field of psychoanalysis has produced a perspective which maintains theoretical integrity but widens its lens to incorporate relational and contextual wisdom. Alternately called a model, field theory, orientation, hybrid, and paradigm, most relational writers have taken pains to indicate that their conceptualizations are based on and incorporate earlier psychodynamic theories. The relational paradigm is a "diverse collection of varied psychoanalytic conceptualizations" (Boston Change Process Study Group, 2013, p. 746) crossing theoretical lines (Harris, 2010), including those of ego psychology, self-psychology, object relations, intersubjectivity (Spezzano, 1998), and attachment theory (DeBei & Dazzi, 2014). As it is referred to in this work, relational analytic theory seeks to utilize preexisting psychodynamic theory as a foundation from which to focus on the processes and dynamics occurring within the therapy relationship.

The relational principles introduced here assume, within their definitions and working formulations, basic psychoanalytic concepts such as internalization of objects, splitting, transference and countertransference, projective identification, and countertransference as non-verbal communication. At key points, the differences between these traditional perspectives and that of relational analytic theory are highlighted. Relational authors, principles, and concepts are directly referenced in this chapter but the psychoanalytic theories from which they are derived are not specified or referenced.

The Beginnings

The roots of relational analytic theory are found in the works of W.R.D. Fairbairn (1952/1996), Sándor Ferenczi (1911/1994a, 1931/1994b), and Harry Stack Sullivan (1965). Fairbairn was a Scottish object relationist, the first to break with drive theory and state that the infant is not pleasure seeking but object seeking. Ferenczi was an early adherent to Freud's theories but split from him over relational issues. He did not agree that analysts should be "blank slates" or that this stance was even possible, nor did he share Freud's conception of the analyst as an objective authority figure who said little. He wrote about the necessity of engaging emotionally with the patient. Sullivan was an early proponent of the interpersonal school and focused on the therapeutic relationship with the psychotic and schizophrenic patients he spent his career treating.

Stephen Mitchell (1988, 2000) is credited with creating our current model of relational analytic thought. He began his writings by critiquing drive theory as missing a relational link and utilized Loewald's theories to develop his system of concepts. Other notable relational writers include Adrianne Harris, Donnel Stern, Jessica Benjamin, and Philip Bromberg.

Core Principles

Relational analytic theory differs from the traditional because it "situates relationship with others at the center of psychic life" (Safran & Kraus, 2014, p. 386). The mental processes of the individual do not occur solely within the boundaries of that individual. All psychic development across the lifespan occurs within a relational context (Russell, 2006). Attachments with others create internalized self-states born of identification with those attachment figures (Mitchell, 2000). This process occurs at a macro as well as a microlevel.

Individuals, their significant others, their families, their neighborhoods, their cultures, and their society are all powerfully interdependent (Harris, 2010). This stance has obvious implications for the therapy relationship.

Here, the patient–therapist relationship is at the center of treatment (Safran & Kraus, 2014). While relational therapy certainly addresses the issues and problems that bring clients to treatment, it prioritizes what unfolds between therapist and client. At some level, this concept is echoed in mainstream treatment. Most practice of psychotherapy accepts that the relationship between client and therapist is the primary mechanism of change (for example, Edwards & Bess, 1998). Furthermore, psychotherapy research consistently demonstrates that the quality of the therapeutic alliance is one of the better predictors of outcome across a range of different treatments, even among those that do not directly address it. No matter what type of therapy offered, unresolved treatment ruptures lead to poor outcome and premature termination (Miller, Luborsky, Barber & Docherty, 1993; Safran & Kraus, 2014).

Several of its principles establish relationally based therapy as unique among the psychodynamic therapies. The first is that therapy is construed as mutually determined, emanating from the conscious and unconscious processes of both parties. Traditional definitions of transference and countertransference are understood as emanating from the client's unconscious issues and relational patterns. In relationally based therapy, the personality of the therapist is as integral to the treatment as is that of the client. Here, engagement, processing, understanding, and behavior all occur through a joint consciousness (Spezzano, 1998). In this constructivist view, meaning is not predetermined but instead created in a dynamic, ongoing manner through dialogue (Benjamin, 2009; Stern, 2010). This co-created dynamic process is at the core of the working alliance.

The second principle is that this joint consciousness produces change. The process of learning to relate with each other while discussing and exploring intimate subjects fuels psychological growth for the client and is "a crucial source of therapeutic action" (Bass, 2003, p. 658). Hence, the third principle is that the relationship itself becomes the primary object of therapeutic scrutiny (Holmes, 2011). Two relational processes in particular, dissociation and enactment, both simultaneously creative and disruptive influences, are the main forces which propel the client and therapist into the change process. Dissociation as a theoretical construct and as applied developmentally to identity formation is presented in this chapter. Because enactment is specific to the therapy process, it is presented and explored in Chaps. 6 and 7 in Part II of the book which is devoted to practice.

Dissociation can be defined as "the separation of mental and experiential contents that would normally be connected" (Howell, 2005, p. 18) or "the ability of the human mind to adaptationally limit its self-reflective capacity" (Bromberg, 1998, p. 7). Trauma theory defines dissociation as a pathological defense mechanism associated with Post Traumatic Stress Disorder. From a relational perspective, dissociation is a normal process powering multiple self-states and shifting states of identity (Harris, 2010). Yet, clearly there is a continuum involved. In normal dissociation, diverse selves and self-states are brought forth in response to varied types of relationships and environments. For example, people utilize different self-states at work than they do when they are parenting at home. This is a healthy process, one that is necessary to fully functional adulthood.

However, other forms of dissociation are less healthy for example, the common experience of missing one's exit off the highway due to "daydreaming" or altered consciousness. When this happens, we do not crash the vehicle because some aspects of our mind remain focused on the task at hand. However, the mental processing which keeps track of the intended exit is "offline." Although this experience is not hazardous, it is disturbing as it occurs outside of our conscious choice (and may make us late).

More potentially dangerous are self-states formed and internalized through neglectful or abusive relationships. At the extreme end of the continuum is dissociation experienced as a result of Dissociative Identity Disorder (DID), where self-states are rigidly and compellingly at odds with each other. In this case, there is no overall observing conscious awareness. When in one self-state, a person with DID does not know of the existence of the others.

As complex human beings however, we are not wholly located at one sole point on the dissociation continuum. We have accrued a multitude of selves over time created as a product of identification with significant others, some healthy and fully evident, others transient, and others hidden from conscious view. Some of these selves are congruent with each other while some are in conflict. With sufficient disparity and incongruence among them, we form symptoms, behave in ways we wish we would not, and engage in predictably rigid and unsatisfying relationships with others.

The two critical factors in assessing the health of a dissociative process are its conscious accessibility and level of flexibility. In normal dissociative self-states, we are aware of our other selves. They function to produce a larger sense of self-coherence; the parts connect together to form a cohesive whole (Harris, 2010). These states are fluid. They shift and transform effortlessly as a given relationship or as situation demands.

Stern (2010) defined pathological dissociation relationally as functioning as a defense mechanism to ward off unformulated self-states, those estranged from thought or language and composed of painful affects, memories, or experiences. He said that "one must not be the person to whom that thing happened, the person who has the feelings, memories, or experiences that come with being that person" (p. 13). Sullivan (1965) deemed the experience of these states as "not-me" and as such, they have not been articulated or verbalized, even within oneself.

When self-states are split off from conscious awareness, memories of events and experiences, cognitions, and affects associated with a specific self-state are unavailable to the overall sense of self. In this case, there are two ways in which the dissociated material can be brought to consciousness and communicated: by suddenly switching into this self-state and thereby losing the rest of the one's sense of self; or in relationship, by enactment. An example of switching from one self-state to another is someone who is alcoholic and who wakes up every morning determined not to drink that day. The addictive self-state is experienced as "not-me." As the day progresses and he becomes increasingly frustrated and distressed, he suddenly decides he is going to drink once finished with his work day. The frustration and distress melt away as the sober self is now experienced as "not-me". This "not-me" process is applicable to multiple stages of this complex struggle illustrated here as a simple duality.

It is important to distinguish this definition of dissociation from the traditional understanding of repression. Although they may appear similar in function in that unmanageable affects are not consciously experienced, the relational model's concept of dissociation involves a vertical split in the mental structure, a departure from Freud's horizontal structure (Harris, 2010; Stern, 2010). Freud's id, ego, and superego are visualized as horizontal layers with the repression barrier maintaining the separation between conscious ego and superego functioning and the id's unconscious repository.

Dissociation, on the other hand, disconnects whole swaths of personality organization, sometimes creating a parallel and co-existing self-state where a system of thoughts, feeling, and behavior is split off from other selves (Goldberg, 2013). While repression functions as a defense serving to maintain the personality system in its entirety, dissociation cuts off conscious connection between separately functioning self-states. These vertical splits prevent the freedom to think and to feel (Stern, 2010), and severely limit self-reflective capacity (Bromberg, 1998) necessary to observe and assess oneself. Since exiling painful affects and experiences renders them unable to be consciously accessed, they remain rigidly constructed. These "not-me" self-states are thus cut off from human relatedness (Bromberg, 1998) and invariably, it is this warded off mental material that produces interpersonal conflict (Holmes, 2011).

Dissociation and Its Impact on Identity Formation: The Descent into Crime

Trauma of all types including those emanating from SES-based experiences? can produce pathological self-states (Harris, 2010) such as the potentially harmful impacts of being raised in poverty and marginalized from the larger society. In an early paper, Mitchell (1993) proposed that chronic aggressive behavior emanates from a self-state of chronic threat and danger. He said that the aggression-based physiological changes causes can disorganize mental processing thereby preventing integration with other self-states. Hence, it is imperative to take into account clients' relationships with their community, culture, and the larger socio-political system in which they live in order to understand how they came to embrace such a destructive lifestyle.

A Cautionary Word About Cause and Effect

Criminologists have developed many divergent sociological and psychological theories to explain the developmental pathways that can lead to a life of crime. The following explanation of the role that trauma and dissociation play in the development of criminal identity and behavior is but one possibility. Popular alternative frameworks are Social Bonds (Hirschi, 1969); Differential Association (Sutherland, 1947; Warr, 1993); and Cognitive Transformation Theory (Maruna, 2001). Other fields have produced studies as well seeking to determine the causes of crime.

For example, current neurobiological research has discovered a correlation between traumatic brain injury (TBI) and antisocial behavior, as TBI can interfere with the modulation of aggression, judgment, and impulse control. Farrer and Hedges (2011) found that, compared with the general population, a significant percentage of those incarcerated suffered serious brain injuries as children. Researchers have discovered that severe child abuse and neglect may cause a hemispheric brain imbalance associated with greater left hemisphere dysfunction and which can lead to antisocial behavior (Walsh & Wu, 2008). Hence, Pemmet (2013) refers to antisocial behavior associated with TBI as acquired sociopathy. Neurobiological research also indicates an association between substance abuse and TBI (McKinlay, Corrigan, Horwood, & Fergusson, 2014).

However, a correlation among factors does not determine causation. Dissociation is a normal mental process. Many children are raised in dysfunctional households or suffer brain injuries, through playing sports for example. It is unfair to equate traumatic upbringings and severe dissociative processes with adult lives of substance abuse, crime, and antisocial behavior. Many, many people raised in traumatic environments have worked hard to overcome the difficulties created by those families and have succeeded in achieving full, successful, and thoroughly prosocial lives.

Similarly, dissociation and its role in identity formation is not the only means with which to understand respondents' trajectories. The focus of this study was not to understand how young men enter a life of crime; it was to discover how they attained and maintained desistance from this life course. Specifically, it explored the impact of their relationships on their desistance processes. But even within this relatively narrow window of study, there are many frameworks that could be appropriately applied for data analysis purposes. I sought one that spoke to me, that could be easily applied to treatment relationships, and that I have applied in my own work. Perhaps as readers consider these ideas, other means and methods with which to study narrative data about desistance will emerge. One of my hopes in writing this book is to spur further research into this area employing this underutilized methodology.

The Developmental Formation of Identity

There are several concepts basic to the relational psychodynamic model which are particularly relevant to the identity formation process explored in this chapter, specifically, the self as formed by interaction with others, dissociation as a psychological defense designed to ward off unformulated affect, and mental organization determined by self-states. Therefore, a brief description of normal identity development based on object relations and attachment theories' principles of attachment, adequate parenting, and identification is presented. The impact of traumatic relationships, environments, and experiences is discussed with special attention paid to the role of parental abuse and neglect in the growing child's developing sense of identity. Respondents' narratives pertaining to the evolution of their criminal identities are examined from this perspective.

Healthy Identity Development

The internal structures of the personality are formed as result of interaction with parental figures in early attachment-based relationships. Beginning in infancy, attachment to caregivers results in a primary identification with them (Balint, 1969/1979). (The terms 'parent' and 'caregiver' are used interchangeably throughout this chapter.) Because infants' interpersonal boundaries have not yet developed, they are not able to distinguish themselves as separate beings from those providing their care. Aspects of parents and caregivers are therefore directly assimilated or incorporated. Along with genetic and constitutional attributes, they become the core of the infants' emerging personality structure (Srinath, 1998).

Modulation of the child's affect is a primary task of early parenting (DeBei & Dazzi, 2014). Infants have limited ability to communicate their needs or tolerate their feeling states. They cry whether they are hungry, wet, cold, in pain or discomfort, scared, or sleepless. When caregivers can accurately assess the cause of the distress and supply adequate food, clothing, and physical care, as well as verbal, emotional, and physical affection, infants learn that their internal states can be soothed from the outside. The world is experienced as a place where their needs may be painful but they are attended to and discomfort is alleviated. It is safe to grow.

As babies develop into toddlers, their capacities for interpersonal boundaries begin to take shape and they become able to distinguish themselves from their caregivers. As a result, the identification process with parents evolves beyond the initial basis of primary identification, characterized by the unmitigated dependency of the infant, to one based on the qualities of the parent–child relationship. Parental traits, capacities, values, and behavior are internalized and assimilated into the developing child's character. As children begin to interact with their outside environments and communities, additional identifications are created from experiences with other adults, such as family members, teachers, clergy, and from relationships with their peers. "We discover ourselves through the images that we perceive in the eyes and looks of others, seeing ourselves in others and finding ourselves in the process" (Srinath, 1998, p. 140).

Emotionally salient interactions with significant others form patterns of experience and of feeling, thinking, and behaving that coalesce into identifications (Stern, 2010). A character structure begins to form from these disparate identifications and a personal sense of agency develops as the child learns to navigate through his or her environment (Temple, 1998). As children approach adolescence, they struggle to develop a cohesive sense of self. Identity coalesces during early adulthood but continues to evolve throughout the entire lifespan (Erikson, 1959/1980).

Parental Abuse and Neglect

All children experience the ebbs and flows of family life. Caregivers cannot always answer immediately. Arguments, discord, and sometimes emergencies occur. As long as parents are capable of overseeing these events and children are not overwhelmed by their distress or left to manage on their own, and absent congenital or hereditary deficits, permanent damage does not occur (Fonagy et al., 1997). However, when parents fail to offer adequate care or when caregivers willfully abuse children, the identificatory system of incorporation and internalization which forms character is gravely affected. In neglectful relationships, parents are too overwhelmed by their own problems and pathology to attend to the child. In abusive relationships, caregivers use the bond to manipulate the child in order to meet their own needs. Often, a neglectful parent enables another caregiver to abuse the child, compounding the damage.

Additionally, abuse can be perpetrated by family members who are not direct caregivers such as siblings and other relatives, or members of the community including other children or adults in positions of authority. The salient factor in these situations is not as much the action taken against the child as it is the parental response to those actions (Harris, 2010). If children trust their parents, they will tell them what happened. If parents believe their children and respond appropriately for the child's benefit rather than based on their own reactions, the experience will have far fewer long-term effects on the child. However, abuse outside the home is far more likely to occur in neglectful households in which children cannot trust their parents to protect them, defend them, or advocate for them.

Children must continue to rely on caregivers whether or not those adults are capable of providing adequate nurture. They do not yet have the resources to self-soothe or take care of themselves. Infant-based attachment is already in place and primary identification has already occurred. Children must maintain the attention and affection of the abusive or neglectful caregiver no matter what the consequences or dreaded experiences. Therefore, they are forced to organize themselves around meeting the needs of the parent in order to get their own needs met (Temple, 1998).

Normal developmental processes yield to the maintenance of the relationship with the abusive or neglectful parent as it is most important to the child's continued functioning. Children have to learn to keep their hand on the proverbial hot stove. Although it is instinctive to yelp in pain and jerk the hand away, they must maintain a connection to the object that continues to cause pain and damage. (For a compelling discussion of these experiences based on analytic concepts, see Eigen, 2001 and Shengold, 1989.)

Dissociation and the Development of Traumatized Self-States

In order to avoid mental disintegration, the child employs psychological defenses to ward off the overwhelming feelings and experience of powerlessness that emanate from this undertaking. One of the defensive methods commonly used is dissociation, "an adaptive and necessary response for the trauma victim" (Davies & Frawley, 1994, p. 41). Dissociation serves two vital functions: first, it permits the child to maintain parts of him or herself as mentally distinct from the pain. The overwhelming anguish is no longer consciously experienced. It becomes "not-me." Parental abuse or neglect that is overwhelming to accept becomes "not them." Simultaneously, however, dissociated self-states also serve to maintain attachment to the abusing or neglectful parent (Bromberg, 1998). Each self-state that disconnects overwhelming and unformulated affect from the conscious personality simultaneously represents the internalization of aspects of the abusive relationship with the caregiver (Davies & Frawley, 1994) creating "false continuities and coherences" to maintain attachments while being traumatized (Harris, 2010, p. 713).

As abusive experiences continue, separate self-states, composed of painful identifications with aspects of caregivers, are spun off. When these self-states are ejected from conscious awareness, all mental processes associated with a specific self-state are unavailable to the overall sense of self. Hence, multiple dissociated states produce a limited conscious awareness, preventing the ability to fully think or feel (Stern, 2010). Whenever unformulated material is triggered by a current situation, demand, or event, dissociated self-states shift in an effort to protect the person from mental disorganization (Bromberg, 1998). And because these states are not conscious or connected with each other, the identifications they hold are fragmented, contradictory, extreme, and frozen: inaccessible to each other and excluded from the maturational processes of the conscious self (Davies & Frawley, 1994).

Traumatized self-states in children can be withdrawn, aggressive, and/or alienated in nature and shift abruptly in response to external events. Internal life may feel chaotic and terrifying, yet conversely, empty. Children may perceive themselves as hurtling through life, bouncing from one situation or relationship to another in a desperate maneuver to avoid their internal states like a pinball driven by the vagaries of their environment.

The defensive use of dissociation interferes with normal mental processing at any point during the lifespan but it causes particular damage during childhood, adolescence, and young adulthood due to the complex developmental demands of growth and maturation (Davies & Frawley, 1994). Children must learn to walk, talk, interact with their families and their peers, function in school, and make sense of themselves and the world around them. The demands of identity formation during adolescence and young adulthood cannot be met through this compromised system. A cohesive identity never starts to form (Holmes, 2011) resulting in identity diffusion, or the inability to integrate contradictory internalizations of self and other (Davies & Frawley, 1994). When consciousness is so fragmented and fragile, it is impossible to understand or articulate the reasons for one's own behavior. It is also impossible to engage in any sustained effort in life or to be emotionally present in close relationships (Bromberg, 1998; Holmes, 2011; Stern, 2010). In other words, healthy growth is unachievable.

Abusive Identifications

The demands of adolescent identity formation place abused children in a quandary. As they begin to experience themselves and others as autonomous individuals, early abusive relationships and traumatic environments impose a dichotomy onto the identity formation process. The growing child can perceive him or herself either as a victim or a victimizer. At this stage of development, there is no in between. Eventually, one or the other of these sets of states predominates within the child's character (Davies & Frawley, 1994) and solidifies into an identificatory system.

At one extreme, children can identify with the victim. For these children, any identification with the aggressor must be consciously disavowed as the victimizer is responsible for causing the pain. The only alternative is to identify with the victim. Yet each self-state dissociated due to abuse has internalized attitudes and aspects of the abuser's character and therefore, they maintain an attachment to the abuser. Hence, even those children who identify with the victim will behave in the manner in which they were treated. They do not act aggressively toward others because they consciously do not want to victimize others. The identification with the abuser is maintained through the child's merciless emotional and physical self-abuse (Davies & Frawley, 1994).

At the other extreme, children who grow up to lead a life of crime have predominant self-states that identify with the aggressors within their families and communities. They experience themselves as being in control when they victimize others (Ganzer & Ornstein, 2008). Mitchell (1993) stated that aggression is a central organizing mechanism of dissociated self-states and by aggressive actions, those who identify with the aggressor disavow the "not-me" states of terror, fear of abandonment, helplessness, and vulnerability created when they were victimized. However, victimizing others causes self-states holding unformulated affect associated with having been victimized to erupt into consciousness. Often, offenders turn to the use of substances to blunt the effect of the suddenly conscious distress.

Trauma and Dissociation in Respondents' Stories

All of the study respondents described traumatic childhoods which would potentially produce severely dissociated self-states. Seven of the 11 respondents were raised in urban ghettoes. Most respondents were children during the 1970s, when life in the ghettoes of major urban cities was precarious and comparable to surviving in a war zone: severe poverty, decrepit housing, abandoned and decaying buildings, addiction, unemployment, familial chaos, and crime rates that were triple or quadruple our current levels. Brother Nowapo's early life sounded as if it were the most extreme. Living in the ghetto of a major city, he witnessed his father's murder as a child. Several other family members were murdered during his early childhood. Jay, Black, Ace, Pink Panther, Mark, and Lee were raised in ghettoes of smaller cities. There, they also described impoverished surroundings and perilous conditions.

Black recounted the conclusion he reached as a teen to identify with the aggressor in response to his chronic sense of vulnerability:

A: I been around violence pretty much my whole life, as a teenager, growing up, even to come outside you'd get picked on, you had to be able to fight back
Q: Defend yourself
A: Yeah, right, so it was just seeing so much violence, it was easy for me to just instead of being a victim, be the victimizer, you know so instead of being hurt, I'd rather hurt first.

Ace described himself as "the black sheep" from a family of achievers. Jay described that his self-state of being a career criminal was produced from his sense of alienation from the larger community:

> As I was doing it [being a career criminal], it became a thing. It was those who was with me in the same mindset. It's us against the world. So all of these people over here are assholes because they're saying this or that … then that's how I was thinking and that's how I was justifying continuing that type of behavior. And it was no problem. I didn't even really think about assaulting someone or robbing someone.

Mark had been abandoned by his father at a very young age. He described that his mother beat him in an attempt to force him to go to school and participate in his education. Mark's early experience of sexual abuse marred his later relationships with women. He said as a young teen, he would engage in relationships with older women and would become violent with them. When I responded to this description by saying that he was being molested, he looked at me blankly and ascribed his treatment of women solely to modeling his behavior after older peers and relatives. Mark was not consciously aware that he was re-creating his sexual abuse by identifying with the aggressor in his intimate relationships. In treating what he considered to be his older girlfriends violently, he was no longer the helpless little boy being sexually abused.

Those respondents who described a less severe environment were still traumatized by abusive families. Bama and Nick were raised in poverty but outside of urban ghettoes by parents who were mentally ill or addicted. Bama said nothing about his early life other than that he grew up around alcohol and drugs, a description curiously absent of people. However, he did describe his relationship with the police. He said, "I grew up where if the police pulled up, you ran whether you done anything or not."

Nick's mother suffered from severe and persistent mental illness and he was sexually and physically abused by one of his brothers. In describing the situation that led to his only arrest and incarceration, he said that his girlfriend, in her teens at the time, had gotten her wisdom teeth removed earlier that day. She was in pain and her face badly swollen. Nick said that he was walking with his girlfriend and that a man had gotten into an altercation with her, hitting her in the jaw. Nick, who was 19 at the time, did not hesitate to punch him three times. Nick had no criminal record at the time but was incarcerated because he violated a law which mandates incarceration for elder abuse as his victim was over 60 years old. Nick identified with the victim in jumping to his girlfriend's defense, associating this assault with his experience at the hands of his older brother but in assaulting a much older and vulnerable man, he identified with the aggressor and behaved in the way his brother once had toward him.

Dee and E described a middle-class upbringing marred by physical abuse, neglect, and mental illness. Dee said he was physically abused by one of his older brothers who also abused many children in the neighborhood. He stated that this abuse accounted for his lifelong anger and aggression.

Dee described situations where his female friends would tell him that they were being abused by their boyfriends. Dee would transform into an avenging angel, arriving on the scene to stop his friend from being bullied or physically hurt. A majority of his arrests began with this scenario. Dee described a shifting of self-states, suddenly losing his ability to pay attention to anything else. It did not matter if he was at work; he would leave to rescue his friend, much in a way that he wished someone would have rescued him from his abusive brother and his own abusive relationships. In an identificatory process similar to that described by Nick, his identification with the victim caused him to leap to his friend's defense. Yet, in doing so, he was unaware of his identification with the aggressor in his response to the situation. He became a neighborhood bully as his brother once was.

E's dissociation was evident throughout his account of his childhood. He described the events of his early life in a flat and emotionless tone. The severe physical abuse E experienced at the hands of his mother, starving him and breaking his fingers, coincided with his early fascination with violence but he was not conscious of the connection between his violent behavior and his identification with his mother's behavior toward him. Nor was he conscious of his father's neglect. Despite his statement that he "started getting diagnosed with things" as a youngster, E consistently denied the impact of his mother's abuse and father's abandonment and neglect on him.

Addiction

In addition to dissociation of self-states, drugs and alcohol provide another powerful means with which to moderate or block overwhelming and unformulated affect. Substance abuse can be embedded in specific self-states (Rothschild & Gellman, 2009) and chronic substance abuse can become its own dissociated identity (Goldberg, 2013) as it requires significant lifestyle and behavioral changes. The chronic substance abusing identity and victimizing self-states can easily subsume each other as they are each defending against the same unformulated material with similar sets of behaviors.

Respondents described a connection between their addicted and violent self-states. Both Lee and Bama maintained how different they were under the influence of substances versus when sober. Lee said he would fight only when drunk. He described it as not being in his "right mind." Bama stated adamantly that he did not have a violent nature. He said he would only behave violently under the influence of alcohol. Despite both respondents' insistence that the substance abusing violent self-state was not their true nature, they spent far more time consciously within these states, behaving in ways they insisted were "not-me."

Dee described a long employment history as a competent restaurant manager yet he could not maintain jobs due to his chronic substance abuse and aggression toward others. He did not associate his substance abuse with his aggressive behaviors despite their co-occurrence. Mark said his criminal self-state never quite fit him. He reported being scared of what he was doing so he would rely on substances as chemical courage.

Respondents also described substance abuse as interfering with their close relationships. Bama was unable to articulate his shifting self-states from sobriety and connectedness with others to solitary alcohol use beyond referring to it as "having rabbit in me." He said he would stay until:

> Got tired of it. Packed my bag and cowed out again. It's what I done for most of my life. Even if I did meet somebody or whatever, it's not a good thing but it wasn't nothin' for me just to go to the store and never come back. Leave everything. Just leave with what I had on.
>
> Q: What would happen to your attachment to those people?
>
> A: (Long pause) I guess, you know, some, eh, I would be drinking when I'd leave. The only time
> I would leave is if I was drunk and I'd say, 'Oh, the hell with it.' I never really got that attached.

Ace said he became addicted to drugs due to an intimate relationship. He said he either "had to do it or leave her and I needed someone to hang on to." Lee stated that his substance abuse was often precipitated by the beginning of an intimate relationship with someone in early recovery. Neither of them able to cope with the demands of an intimate relationship, they would both undo each other's attempts at sobriety.

Turning Points

Continued failure in life after the development of dissociated self-states in childhood causes overwhelming frustration and despair, often leading to more unformulated affective responses which then require more dissociation. It is a system of increasing pathology and diminishing returns. As Jay spent more and more time with his addicted self-state consciously in control, his life became more and more restricted. Looking back from a period of secondary desistance, he described himself as feeling "boxed in." Eventually, he was facing a life sentence. Dee said he was increasingly angry at the world and angry at himself. E described an identity devoted to ineffective treatment attempts, describing himself as a "professional client." Mark realized as he was facing his first incarceration that his lifestyle had become unmanageable. Ace said after multiple detox attempts that "three strikes and I was out."

Turning points occurred in each of the study respondents' lives in which they were able to observe and assess their criminal and substance abusing self-states. Although they could not have articulated the correlation among attachment, identification, identity, and behavioral change, they realized that changing their lives required fundamentally different relationships with people. They described knowing that they had to form attachments to those outside of a criminal and substance abusing lifestyle. They had to let go of the mistrust of members of the larger community and begin to seek their help, guidance, and support in order to change their lives and the trajectory of their paths.

References

Altman, N. (2005). Psychoanalysis and the urban poor. In L. Aron & A. Harris (Eds.), *Relational psychoanalysis: Volume 2 innovation and expansion*. Hillsdale, NJ: Analytic Press.

Balint, M. (1979). *The basic fault*. New York: Brunner/Mazel. (Original work published 1969).

Bass, A. (2003). "E" Enactments in psychoanalysis: Another medium, another message. *Psychoanalytic Dialogues, 13*, 657–675.

Benjamin, J. (2009). Psychoanalytic controversies: A relational psychoanalysis perspective on the necessity of acknowledging failure in order to restore the facilitating and containing features of the intersubjective relationship (the shared third). *International Journal of Psychoanalysis, 90*, 441–450.

Boston Change Process Study Group. (2013). Enactment and the emergence of new relational organization. *Journal of the American Psychoanalytic Association, 61*, 727–749.

Bromberg, P. M. (1998). *Standing in the spaces: Essays on clinical process, trauma, & dissociation*. Hillsdale, NJ/London: Analytic Press.

Davies, J. M., & Frawley, M. G. (1994). *Treating the adult survivor of childhood sexual abuse: A psychoanalytic perspective*. New York: Basic Books.

DeBei, F., & Dazzi, N. (2014). Attachment and relational psychoanalysis. *Psychoanalytic Dialogues, 24*, 562–577.

Edwards, J. K., & Bess, J. M. (1998). Developing effectiveness in the therapeutic use of self. *Clinical Social Work Journal, 26*, 89–106.

Eigen, M. (2001). *Damaged bonds*. New York/London: Karnac.

Erikson, E. H. (1980). *Identity and the life cycle*. New York: W.W. Norton. (Original work published (1959).

Fairbairn, W. R. D. (1996). *Psychoanalytic studies of the personality*. London/New York: Routledge. (Original work published 1952).

Farrer, T. J., & Hedges, D. W. (2011). Prevalence of traumatic brain injury in incarcerated groups compared to the general population: A meta-analysis. *Progress in Neuro-Psychopharmacology & Biological Psychiatry, 35*, 390–394.

Ferenczi, S. (1994a). *First contributions to psycho-analysis*. London: Karnac Books. (Original work published 1911).

Ferenczi, S. (1994b). *Final contributions to the problems and methods of psycho-analysis*. London: Karnac Books. (Original work published 1931).

Fonagy, P., Target, M., Steele, M., Steele, H., Leigh, T., Levinson, A., et al. (1997). Morality, disruptive behavior, borderline personality disorder, crime and their relationship to security of attachment. In L. Atkinson & K. J. Zucker (Eds.), *Attachment and psychopathology* (pp. 223–276). New York/London: The Guilford Press.

Ganzer, C., & Ornstein, E. D. (2008). In and out of enactments: A relational perspective on the short- and long-term treatment of substance abuse. *Clinical Social Work Journal, 36*, 155–164.

Goldberg, A. I. (2013). *Being of two minds: The vertical split in psychoanalysis and psychotherapy*. New York/London: Routledge.

Harris, A. E. (2010). The relational tradition: Landscape and canon. *Journal of the American Psychoanalytic Association, 59*, 701–735.

Hirschi, T. (1969). *Causes of delinquency*. Berkeley, CA: University of California Press.

Holmes, J. (2011). Donnel Stern and relational psychoanalysis. *British Journal of Psychotherapy, 27*, 305–315.

Howell, E. F. (2005). *The dissociative mind*. Hillsdale, NJ/London: Analytic Press.

Maruna, S. (2001). *Making good: How ex-convicts reform and rebuild their lives*. Washington, DC: American Psychological Association.

McKinlay, A., Corrigan, J., Horwood, L. J., & Fergusson, D. M. (2014). Substance abuse and criminal activities following traumatic brain injury in childhood, adolescence, and early adulthood. *Journal of Head Trauma Rehabilitation, 29*, 498–506.

Miller, N. E., Luborsky, L., Barber, J. P., & Docherty, J. P. (1993). *Psychodynamic treatment research: A handbook for clinical practice*. New York: Basic Books.

Mitchell, S. A. (1988). *Relational concepts in psychoanalysis*. Cambridge, MA/London: Harvard University Press.

Mitchell, S. A. (1993). Aggression and the endangered self. *Psychoanalytic Quarterly, 62*, 351–382.

Mitchell, S. A. (2000). *Relationality: From attachment to intersubjectivity*. Hillsdale, NJ: Analytic Press.

Pemmet, J. (2013). Psychopathy versus sociopathy: Why the distinction has become crucial. *Aggression and Violent Behavior, 18*, 458–461.

Rothschild, D., & Gellman, M. (2009). Finding the common ground: Contemporary psychoanalysis and substance abuse treatment. *Journal of Addictive Diseases, 28*, 28–38.

Russell, P. L. (2006). On waiting for the right time. *Smith College Studies in Social Work, 76*, 99–104.

Safran, J. D., & Kraus, J. (2014). Alliance ruptures, impasses and enactments: A relational perspective. *Psychotherapy, 51*, 381–387.

Shengold, L. (1989). *Soul murder: The effects of childhood abuse and deprivation*. New York: Fawcett Columbine.

Spezzano, C. (1998). Listening and interpreting: How relational analysts kill time between disclosures and enactments. *Psychoanalytic Dialogues, 8*, 237–246.

Srinath, S. (1998). Identificatory processes in trauma. In C. Garland (Ed.), *Understanding trauma: A psychoanalytic approach* (pp. 139–154). New York: Routledge.

Stern, D. B. (2010). Partners in thought: Working with unformulated experience, dissociation, and enactment. In D. B. Stern (Ed.), *Psychoanalysis in a new key* (Vol. 12). New York/London: Routledge.

Sullivan, H. S. (1965). *Personal psychopathology: Early formulations*. New York: W.W. Norton & Company.

Sutherland, E. (1947). *Criminology* (4th ed.). New York: Lippincott.

Temple, N. (1998). Developmental injury: Its effects on the inner world. In C. Garland (Ed.), *Understanding trauma: A psychoanalytic approach* (pp. 155–166). New York: Routledge.

Walsh, A., & Wu, H. (2008). Differentiating antisocial personality disorder, psychopathy, and sociopathy: Evolutionary, genetic, neurological, and sociological considerations. *Criminal Justice Studies, 21*, 135–152.

Warr, M. (1993). Parents, peers and delinquency. *Social Forces, 72*, 247–264.

4

Pathways to Desistance

Abstract This chapter presents results of the analysis of respondents' desistance narratives. The process of desistance from criminal behavior and substance abuse was analyzed in terms of the pathways respondents took and how their significant relationships functioned to assist them. Primary desistance, the preliminary attempts at sobriety and curtailing criminal behavior, is distinguished from secondary desistance in which an identity change occurs and all antisocial behavior stops. The types of relationships respondents engaged in and the elements of these relationships crucial to desistance are explored particularly as they impacted new identity formation. Affective, cognitive, and behavioral aspects of this process are described. Identification with others is highlighted as the pivotal mechanism creating the capacity for this transformation. Cultural and societal obstacles to desistance are discussed.

Desistance from criminal behavior and substance abuse is a developmental journey, a complex process achieved over time often comprising several phases and multiple attempts. This chapter furthers the exploration of respondents' narratives, moving from their entry into crime and substance abuse to the course of their progression to desistance, including how their significant relationships functioned to facilitate this life transition. Respondents' primary and

© The Editor(s) (if applicable) and The Author(s) 2016

D.H. Benveniste, *Changing Substance Abuse and Criminal Behavior Through Therapeutic Relationships*, DOI 10.1057/978-1-137-53039-4_4

secondary desistance pathways are described. The types of participants' relationships are presented, their important elements are discussed, and the role each relationship played in the desistance process is explored particularly as it impacted new identity formation. Identification with others is highlighted as the pivotal mechanism creating the capacity for this transformation. Cultural and societal obstacles to desistance are discussed.

Primary and Secondary Desistance Pathways

Criminologists describe two general pathways to desistance. Primary desistance is defined as a latency phase in which serious criminal behavior stops but petty crime continues (Irwin, 1970). These are the preliminary attempts to stop antisocial behavior and substance abuse. Secondary desistance involves an identity shift from criminal to prosocial community member in which all criminal activity ceases (Farrall & Calverley, 2006; Glaser, 1969). This is a far more difficult endeavor as it demands not only changes to behavior but also a profound transformation of the psyche.

Using a visual display based on Saldana's (2013) work, there were three pathways that respondents followed in their desistance process as indicated in Fig. 4.1:

The first two desistance pathways begin with significant relationships and their direct contributions toward secondary desistance. Pathway One

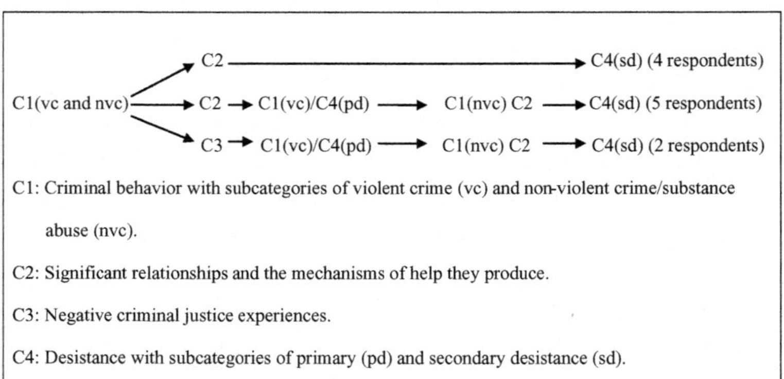

Fig. 4.1 Desistance pathways

avoids primary desistance altogether and moves directly from significant relationships to secondary desistance. Pathways Two and Three include primary desistance but the impetus for this first shift differs.

In the second pathway, primary desistance results from significant relationships and involves the cessation of violent crime while non-violent criminal behavior and substance abuse continue. Significant relationships come into play again to help facilitate the final shift to secondary desistance. In the third pathway, primary desistance results from negative criminal justice (CJ) experiences and involves the cessation of violent crime. Non-violent substance-based criminal behavior continues. Significant relationships help facilitate the final shift to secondary desistance. Table 4.1 presents the secondary desistance pathways reported by all eleven respondents.

Four of the 11 respondents (Nick, Mark, Black, and Jay) followed the first pathway. They did not describe experiencing a primary desistance phase; rather they ceased criminal behavior entirely and all at once. Nick never described himself as identifying as a criminal. Furthermore, his experiences while incarcerated so traumatized him that he decided he would never return. After a long criminal history, Mark reported that he stopped committing crimes after his first arrest leading to an incarceration. Black said that he had spent most of his adult life incarcerated. Once married, however, he reported ceasing all criminal behavior. Jay reported a variety of factors influencing his decision to desist including family members desisting, his mother's death, and facing mandatory sentencing.

The other seven respondents, Lee, E, Bama, Ace, Pink Panther, Brother Nawapo, and Dee, described processes that corresponded to both phases of desistance. For their primary desistance phase, they all reported curtailing violent behavior, the most serious of their offenses. Five respondents, Lee, E, Bama, Brother Nawapo, and Dee, reported that relational experiences facilitated their primary desistance, as indicated by the second pathway. The other two, Ace and Pink Panther, attributed their primary desistance to negative experiences with the CJ system, as indicated by the third pathway. They all then continued with less serious substance abuse-related crime until they achieved secondary desistance, sometimes occurring many years later.

Table 4.1 Respondents' descriptions of their secondary desistance pathways

Pseudonym	Length of time in secondary desistance	Turning points into secondary desistance	Types of behaviors representative of secondary desistance
Nick	11 years	Avoid prison	Friends for support, avoids conflicts, follows therapist's guidance
Black	4 years	Marriage, birth of son, death of mother	Follows wife's guidance, stay-at-home parent
Mark	10 years	Halfway house, SA treatment, children	Working in social services, accepted guidance
Jay	3 years	CJ system, relational experiences, OP SA treatment	HIV sober house, social service job
Pink Panther	5 months	Death of significant other	MH treatment, living on own
Ace	9 years	Family got him to detox	Living on own, AA, MH treatment, volunteer work
Brother Nawapo	2 years	MH and HIV treatment	Self-care, avoids conflicts, ended relationship
Dee	13 months	MH and HIV treatment	Accepting self and guidance re: treatment HIV sober house
Bama	16 months	Girlfriend	Working at AA and relationship
E	5 years	SA treatment	Kept attempting treatment until it "took," parenting
Lee	4 months	Second chance at HIV sober house	Re-establishing relationships with family

Key: *SA* substance abuse, *MH* mental health, *CJ* criminal justice, *OP* outpatient

Table 4.2 presents descriptions of the primary desistance pathways for the seven respondents.

The Role of Significant Relationships in Desistance

All eleven respondents stated that significant relationships were crucial to their successful desistance process. Sampson and Laub (1993, 2003) found that a strong attachment and close emotional ties with non-criminally

Table 4.2 Respondents' descriptions of their primary desistance pathways

Pseudonym	Years in primary desistance	Turning points into primary desistance	Types of behaviors representative of primary desistance
Pink Panther	3.5	Negative CJ system experiences	SA
Ace	11	Negative CJ system experiences	SA, petty crime
Brother Nawapo	3	Sense of self-change re HIV, accepting treatment	First attempt sober house
Dee	5	SA treatment	SA
Bama	9	Positive CJ system relational experiences	Alcohol, hopping trains
E	13	Relational experiences	SA
Lee	3	SA treatment	Alcohol and related incarceration

Key: *SA* substance abuse, *CJ* criminal justice

involved co-workers, bosses, teachers, classmates, or spouses provided effective support for men in the desistance process. The respondents of this study listed three primary types of relationships most helpful to them: (1) those with 12 Step program participants such as AA or NA; (2) those with substance abuse (SA), mental health (MH) treatment, or social services staff; and (3) those with family, including intimate relationships, children, and grandchildren. Each respondent identified relationships with at least three people who played essential roles for them, with an average of five per respondent. Additionally, involvement with the CJ system provided relational impacts for five respondents.

Types of Significant Relationships

Ten of the 11 study respondents listed relationships with those in positions of help: AA/NA members, SA and MH treatment, and general social services as essential to their success. AA/NA relationships occur as a product of AA/NA meetings, are voluntary, and are based on 12 Step principles. MH and SA treatment are provided by paid professionals trained in those fields to help people stabilize their emotional and behavioral lives. Workers providing general social services assist individuals with access to governmental and community entitlements and programs.

These relationships were described as quite diverse in length, some short and others very long term. One respondent described relationships at both ends of the spectrum. Brother Nawapo described a single meeting with a social service worker who was able to discuss his HIV status with him without triggering his rage. She was able to interest him in an out-of-state HIV sober house to which she referred him. He was residing there at the time of the interview. He also described his MH therapist with whom he had been meeting for 3 years as crucial to his recovery.

Two respondents indicated that SA treatment was the primary factor in facilitating their desistance. Lee began to stop his assaultive behavior after his first stint in a sober house and Dee stopped violent behavior after his first attempt at SA treatment. Jay also described attending SA treatment shortly after his most recent release from prison and genuinely participating for the first time.

> Once I got out, I was involved in Narcotics Anonymous. I got really involved. I had a lot of fears, not sharing really what was going on with me, not really talking about real issues, so I knew that I had to do things different than I did before. I would be in a crowd, but I really wouldn't be there before. Now, I will go to meetings, share, and it doesn't really matter what other people think. I remember a guy told me, a director, I was talking to him, and I was always telling him about how I thought other people would think, and he was like, "Wow, man, you know, you should be a multimillionaire if you can think for other people." But that's how it was in my mind. I already knew what you was going to think if I said this or that. And I was in a box, man. I boxed myself in. And that went on for years, man.

Of the ten respondents who identified SA as a problem, nine described relationships with AA/NA as being vital to their ongoing sobriety and desistance from violent behavior. They described the availability of meetings, their routine, other respondents in recovery, and volunteering for coffee-making or cleanup as important features of the ongoing support that AA/NA provides. Four men indicated that it was their sponsors who provided the most important support.

Helpful Elements of Relationships

All study respondents were able to identify aspects from each of their relationships that provided support and how that support then served to reinforce their desistance processes. Ten respondents listed care, nine listed guidance, and all 11 listed both trust and support as crucial aspects of these relationships. One respondent used the term "sense of belonging." Seven listed "never give up" and seven listed "non-judgmental" as features they found necessary in effective helpful relationships.

In addition to the aspects above, respondents also listed the following as important: belief in the interviewee (2), death of a significant relationship (6), encouragement (6), relationships with children or grandchildren (7), reliability (6), others functioning as role models (4), people who help the interviewee set boundaries (2), and wisdom (3).

These factors can be grouped into the following categories. Elements of relationships that are affect- or emotion-based are caring, trust, belief in the respondent, encouragement, never giving up on the respondent, support, and reliability. Cognitive or thought-based elements are guidance, setting boundaries, and being a role model for the respondent. Additionally, the category of changing social relationships—the death of a significant other and relationships with children and grandchildren—includes both affective and cognitive components. Each of the three categories includes items related to the identification process. These groups of factors combined to facilitate respondents' identity and behavioral change.

The Process of Identity Change

Identity is defined as a consistent and coherent sense of who one is (Maruna, 2001). It includes depictions of the self, personal attributes, and social roles and their meanings, highlighting both what we have in common with others and what distinguishes us from other people (Presser, 2008). Most respondents found that in order to fully renounce the lifestyle and subculture that accompanies long-term, serious criminal behavior and substance abuse, an identity shift was necessary.

Nine of 11 study participants described an identity change that occurred as a result of their desistance. Two respondents, Nick and Ace, stated that their identity or sense of themselves as people did not change when they desisted from criminal behavior and substance abuse. At the time of the interviews, both had successfully avoided criminal behavior and been sober for more than a decade.

Nick reported that he committed one violent act when he was an older teenager, did not commit any other crime, and did not have an SA problem. Although Nick described supportive friends who helped him maintain a violence-free lifestyle, he did not describe an identity shift that occurred along with his decision to avoid violent behavior. Nick was raised in the foster care system and was receiving Social Security Disability benefits for mental illness. Based on his narrative, it would appear that his identity derived from his family history of mental illness.

Ace disagreed that he was working to change his identity, saying, "Not my identity, who I am. It's not going to change that." However, he said he was putting 100% into changing his behavior. Everyone else described an identity based on criminal activity or substance abuse that had to be completely transformed in order for them to stop the associated behaviors.

Identification In order to change one's identity, it is necessary to internalize and integrate identifications from relationships with new significant others. A sense of self that supports prosocial behavior derives from two identification processes: the capacity to identify with prosocial people and the ability to identify with others as victims (Farrall & Calverley, 2006; Maruna, 2001). Through these two identificatory processes, the desister increasingly feels that he belongs to the prosocial community, has a role within it, and can see himself differently. As Brother Nawapo and many others described it, their identity becomes that of a productive member of the community.

Respondents described two affective, three cognitive, and one behavioral theme relating to identification. The first affective theme, a non-criminally involved person seeing something good in the respondent and being given a second chance, facilitated the respondent being able to see himself differently, through another's eyes. This experience is a prerequisite to being able to identify with another.

Being Perceived as Good by Non-criminally Involved Others and Being Given a Second Chance All seven studies that explored the mechanisms of social bonds relevant to the desistance process reviewed for this project (Aresti, Eatough, & Brooks-Gordon, 2010; Farrall, 2004;

Haggard, Gumpert, & Grann, 2001; Hughes, 1998; Meisenhelder, 1982; Rains-Russell, 2009; Walker, 2010) confirmed that being perceived as good by prosocial significant others was critical to desistance. The experience of being accepted and valued by prosocial others validates and supports prosocial identity development (Aresti et al., 2010; Maruna, 2001; Meisenhelder, 1982). Eight respondents (Bama, Lee, Jay, Mark, Brother Nawapo, Dee, Black, and Ace) described experiencing a shift in their sense of themselves after being perceived differently by others.

Four of these respondents, Black, Lee, Brother Nawapo, and Bama, mentioned being given second chances as watershed moments. Bama felt this way about the warden who arranged for his parole but he had another positive experience with a representative of the CJ system, his parole officer. He described leaving a halfway house due to deplorable conditions and leaving the state to see his mother, both in violation of his parole. He said he had made several attempts to inform his parole officer about the condition of the halfway house prior to departing, to no avail.

When Bama returned and presented himself to his parole officer, he fully expected his parole to be violated. Instead, his parole officer investigated the halfway house and shut it down. Bama said that both the warden and his parole officer saw something in him that he had not seen in himself. He described that this experience changed Bama's perception, both of himself and about the representative of the CJ system who trusted Bama's word instead of reacting based on the rules.

Brother Nawapo talked about being readmitted to the residential program where he was residing at the time of the interview. He reported that he had had "an altercation" with the former program director and had to leave but was readmitted by the current director. He described her as "much more humble, much more caring, much more considerate" and said, "She hasn't passed judgment on me yet and the way she carries herself is very professional." Brother Nawapo was describing that the new director cared about him, believed in him, and was encouraging him to try again, all affective interventions.

The Impact of Younger Family Members Several of the studies reviewed for this project underscored the importance of family in desisters' lives, specifically the role of their children (Bahr, Harris, Fisher, & Armstrong, 2010; Farrall & Calverley, 2006; Hughes, 1998; Walker, 2010). Hughes (1998) stated that perhaps as a result of their own impoverished childhoods, her respondents understood the vital role parents play in their children's lives. This second affective theme not only allowed respondents to see themselves through the eyes of their younger family members but also permitted them to understand the pain they caused to their children by their own behavior.

Mark, Lee, Jay, Ace, Black, and E described their sense of themselves change in response to younger family members' emotional needs. Mark reported being determined to raise his youngest children "from birth to death" and to be the father to them that he himself never had. Lee's intention was to be there for his son's children to make amends for not being there for his son. These respondents described experiencing the process of identifying with another person's emotional pain and sought to avoid recreating those conditions for those relying on them.

Jay and Ace talked about the importance of feeling that they were role models for younger cousins and nieces. Black attributed his desistance entirely to his relationships with his wife and son. He described that his source of self-esteem derives from being a good husband and father. E described the change in how he viewed himself once his son was born. He said, "My son is the second best thing I have ever done in my life." (The first was achieving sobriety.) He added, "For the first time in my life, I am okay with E."

Changes in Negative Perceptions of Others A cognitive theme presented by respondents is the ability to view members of the larger society, particularly representatives of the CJ system and other authority figures, in a non-negative light. Byrne and Trew (2008) found in their study of ex-offenders that those who reoffended maintained their negative stance toward formal social institutions including the CJ and treatment systems. Successful desisters changed their views.

Four respondents, Dee, Bama, Jay, and Brother Nawapo, reported changing their perceptions of others. These shifts occurred due to positive emotional experiences with new prosocial significant others. Dee said he stopped caring what others thought about his HIV status and sexual orientation once he began treatment at a sober house for people who are HIV+ and felt an experience of belonging. He said that he could then relate to people and stop running from his illness. Bama stated:

> Over so many years, you got your idea of people. So when somebody else goes against that, what you're thinking, it's kinda suspicious but actually you see that there's no catch to it. They just want you to do good.

A similar change of perception was experienced by eight respondents, Nick, Jay, Black, E, Brother Nawapo, Lee, Bama, and Dee, who described learning the ability to positively utilize familial attachments no matter how negative some of their childhood experiences may have been. Bahr et al. (2010) found that those respondents who experienced their families as more of a stress than a resource were more likely to recidivate. They viewed their families as dysfunctional and demanding rather than as helpful which created obstacles to desistance.

These eight respondents who described stressful family situations were able to reframe their experiences in a positive light. For example, although his family did not provide him with any typical avenues of support, Nick stated that he received services at two MH agencies which provided many concrete services, particularly helpful to him as he was homeless. He related that his mother used to bring him to these agencies when he was a child so he both knew about them and was known to them when he needed their services later in life. It is possible that as respondents were able to see themselves in a more positive light, their views of their families' efforts improved as well.

Death of a Significant Other The death of a significant other was a more complex experience for respondents. Five study participants, E, Pink Panther, Black, Ace, and Jay, indicated that it was the loss of people important to them which provided the main impetus for entering primary desistance. Although the death of a significant other would normally be categorized as an emotional experience due to feelings of loss, it is included here as additionally affecting cognition because respondents reported primarily positive cognitive impacts.

The common factor of these stories is that although this significant other cared deeply for the respondent, he or she was not able to provide guidance while alive. The loss of this person forced changes in introspection, self-perception, and behavior. In contrast, qualitative studies reviewed for this study did not indicate deaths of significant others as important positive factors in respondents' desistance processes. E related that being told of his father's terminal illness while he was incarcerated served as the motivation for him to stop engaging in violent behavior:

> So I get out from there [prison] and some things happened while I was in. I was confronted with the thought of my father dying. And he made a specific point of driving down from [state where he lived] to look me in the eye and tell me that he was not proud of me and I wasn't the son he had raised. And then he started getting cancer. He got multiple cancers in '99 I think. I went in in like '97. In '99, I committed myself to leading a positive lifestyle even in that environment.

Pink Panther described a long-term and close but dysfunctional relationship with his girlfriend as both were drug-involved. He reported grieving her loss deeply after she passed away but that her death enabled him to stop using and engaging in crime because he was "on his own now" which made him "very independent, more responsible, and a stronger person." He said, "I'm a much better person than to get high because of feelings."

After her death, Pink Panther was able to integrate positive aspects of his attachment to his girlfriend as a part of himself. He said he could no longer see himself as a relapser, stating, "The longer I stay clean, the happier she will be because she sees." Here, Pink Panther utilizes a thought about himself based on his attachment to his girlfriend for affect management purposes in order to avoid using drugs.

Four respondents, Pink Panther, Bama, Jay, and Black, reported that the illness or death of their mothers provided the initial motivation for desistance. They described that their mothers would no longer be there to enable their criminal behavior. Black said:

A: She's passed away now you know, I lost her like three years ago, almost four years ago—actually, 2008 in March.
Q: That was close to around the time that you decided to straighten up—
A: Yup, yup. I came home in February, and that was, she died in March—

Q: Did that have anything to do with it?
A: Yeah, I think it did, I think it did. Because you know, I'm the baby and she was like always there for me going to jail. I had commissary. I knew she would come or she always made sure the phone was on for me to call, just those little things you know that everybody's not going to do for you. She never shut me off. She would get tired of my BS but she never gave up on me… I came home and then when she passed, it was like, "I definitely got to do something different!"

Achieving the Capacity to Identify with Others For those who have victimized others, the capacity to identify with other people is crucial to the desistance process (Pithers, 1990). It provides the basis upon which affective and cognitive processes consolidate to change behavior. The ability to comprehend that the offender experiences the same type of emotional and physical pain as is caused to others by his antisocial acts provides a strong motivation to avoid doing harm and to engage in prosocial behaviors. Without being able to perceive others as having the same needs and feelings as himself, a person may avoid violence or substances due to external pressures such as fear of job loss or restrictions to movement like incarceration. However, any change based on external repercussions alone will only last as long as those factors are present.

Farrall and Calverley (2006) described their respondents as experiencing feelings of guilt and shame when contemplating a return to criminal behavior because of the impact on the victim. Seven respondents (Dee, Jay, Pink Panther, Mark, E, Brother Nawapo, and Nick) described a newly formed capacity to identify with others which helped them determine that they wanted to avoid violence. Dee said, "I know how it feels to be beat on. Why would I want to do that to somebody else?" Pink Panther said that he should have known better than to put his hands on his girlfriend. Mark discovered that "it is retarded to keep women by scaring them." He said that he learned to be nice to them instead. Nick talked about learning to be patient with people in order to avoid confrontations. E refers to people who have never had a substance abuse problem or have been in recovery as "civilians." He said he is more tolerant and understanding of them because they do not have the tools that AA has given him.

Work in a Social Service Role Nine respondents worked in or planned to work in the social services. Consistent with the literature (Aresti et al., 2010; Hughes, 1998; Irwin, 1970; Maruna, 2001), they described this activity as crucial to their desistance. Calling it a "generative role" (based on Maruna's [2001] concept of a generative script), Aresti, et al. (2010, p.171) stated that using past experience in working with those in socially excluded groups is an instrumental feature in the shift to a positive self-conception.

Either as volunteer or paid employee, it appears that social services work provided study respondents with three critical functions: a two-pronged means to facilitate and validate an identity shift as well as a means with which to support behavioral change. Being accepted as an employee or volunteer provides a positive sense of self, a sense of belonging, and the feeling that the organization believes in the respondent because he is trusted by influential and prosocial others. Additionally, respondents reported that they were viewed as role models by the recipients of the service, providing another means with which to view themselves differently. They also described feeling an obligation to maintain their sobriety and non-violent behavior as a result of their role model status.

Three respondents, E, Mark, and Jay, are employed in social services. Jay said of his work experience, "If I fail, so will a lot of others." The other two study participants worked for agencies which provided their treatment, E as a program administrator and Mark as a client supervisor in a correctional halfway house. Clearly, hiring a former client indicates a strong endorsement. To progress from service recipient to service provider, to view staff as role models and then become one himself, serves as a significant and positive emotional experience and requires the internalization of some of the staff's values and perceptions.

Mark had two other part-time jobs as a home health aide. E and Jay were volunteers in addition to their paid employment. Four respondents, Black, Pink Panther, Brother Nawapo, and Ace, volunteered for social service agencies including a homeless shelter, a soup kitchen, and a drop in center for substance abusers. Ace identified a sense of belonging gained from his volunteer work. Brother Nawapo's goal was to become an SA counselor as part of his identification with his MH therapist.

Although Dee and Bama did not report volunteer activities at the time of the interview, Dee said he recently passed his exam to be a certified nurse's aide and was pursuing employment as a CNA. He stated that he chose this field as way to give back to others. He also wanted to study to become an HIV counselor. Bama would give talks at AA meetings about his substance abuse history and recovery to help him maintain his commitment to sobriety and to provide guidance and encouragement to others. Two respondents, Lee and Nick, did not report doing any social service or volunteer work.

Respondents talked about these goals and activities as reinforcing their sense of themselves as better people and more productive members of society. Jay described the impact of his work as a residential aide at a homeless shelter:

A: I love doing it. I didn't know that I have—you know even here, even though I'm not from this area, I have a lot of information that I can help people with. And I used to think before- I remember in [city where he was residing], a lot of the residents would come to me, and I used to go back into that mode of you know, these people think I'm soft. And I remember one of the other staffs telling me the reason they come to you is because they know you're going to treat them right. [Jay chuckled and then started to cry.]
Q: What are the feelings that you have about that? Can you say?
A: Because I've never seen that in myself.

As study respondents experienced these relationships and processes, they reported that they began to sense that something within themselves was changing. Two respondents described their first moments of conscious realization of their shift in identity. Black described returning to the city where he had grown up and saying to himself, "You ain't that dude no more." Jay said, "I remember a lot of times, I would go to jail and get out, and see people that I was right there with. [They] was looking like walking death and I'm like, wow, you know, that was me." Neither Black nor Jay underwent primary desistance. In their discussion of identity change, they are referencing an aspect of secondary desistance.

In addition to themes related to the identification process, there are several other capacities crucial to the transition to desistance. Affect management, the ability to govern negative feeling states, and the ability to accept guidance from others, a cognitive skill, both combine to produce effects on behavior. Additionally, respondents described two capacities they used to control their behavior: being careful when engaging in intimate relationships and making daily conscious decisions to avoid violence and substances.

Affect Management Defined as the ability to experience feelings consciously and express them verbally, affect management enables one to tolerate intense feelings without resorting to impulsive behavioral means with which to alleviate them. Without it, negative self-states comprising frustration, anger, confusion, shame, hostility, or guilt can overwhelm coping mechanisms. In healthy development, affect management is attained through early nurturing experiences with caregivers but those capacities are impaired for those raised in traumatic environments. In this case, the ability to manage one's affect must be incorporated through later relationships with significant others. Through several interlocking mechanisms, interpersonal exchanges with significant others facilitate affect management by reducing the impact of negative self-states.

At the most basic level, in order to communicate one's negative feeling states to another, it is necessary to verbalize the affect. Translating feelings into spoken words requires that they be fully present in one's awareness and not discharged through a dissociative process, use of a substance, or by an impulsive action. This ability is the first step in containing the negative feeling. Respondents then described receiving supportive or encouraging feedback which permitted them to see themselves through the other's eyes, thereby reducing the intensity of the negative self-state.

Once calmer, respondents were able to utilize cognitive skills and guidance offered by their significant other in order to perceive the situation differently. They could then conceptualize different coping strategies or prosocial behaviors with which to respond. As the internal sense of personal agency improved and a feeling of control occurred, the negative self-state was either reduced or eliminated entirely. In some cases, this exchange freed the respondent to experience new thought processes about the causes of the painful states.

Nine respondents, Pink Panther, E, Mark, Brother Nawapo, Nick, Dee, Lee, Jay, and Black, talked about the impact of learning to improve their feeling states and stress tolerance by sharing negative emotions with others. Mark discussed his disclosure of being sexually molested as a child:

> I swore I take that to my grave. Never, never tell another soul and I got to the program and I talked about it and I understood how that incident kind of got in my life to the way it went, too.
>
> But growing up, I never equated anything I did with the really bad things that happened to me.
>
> You know what happened with that girl was something that I never talk about, try not to think about it if I can, and not having a father, now that I talk about it, try not to think about it and I never equated that me going through this with this girl may have caused me along with some of my other teachings to be like I was with women.

Mark described disclosing his abuse after feeling accepted and trusting in his treatment program. This disclosure opened cognitive connections between the loss of his father and being sexually molested as a child with his later abusive and criminal behavior.

E said that he "lets resentment go immediately" and does not engage in self-pity as those are dangerous feelings for him to have. Jay said that he "puts feelings in perspective and moves on." Black stated that he does not keep things "bottled up" and instead tells his wife. He said that she keeps him "focused and grounded."

Lee ascribed most of his success with sobriety to sharing his feelings with others. He reported that he calls his sponsor daily and that he talks to the staff or residents at the sober house in which he resides. He said, "If you let somebody know what goin' on with you, the thought disappears." He said that not holding feelings within himself eliminates his urges to use alcohol. Lee is describing affect management provided by sharing negative feeling states with significant others as having a direct effect on his compulsions to use.

Acceptance of Guidance Once respondents could manage their feelings effectively, they realized that they needed to learn from others how to think and behave differently. Consistent with the literature, all 11 study respondents came to understand that improving self-perception and personal behavior results from accepting the instructions and suggestions of trusted others. Bahr, et al. (2010), Haggard et al. (2001), and Leibrich (1993) emphasized the positive impact of SA and MH treatment on the desistance process. Mark talked about the impact of a halfway house treatment program in which he participated as part of his sentence. He said that he found that his thinking was "all messed up" and learned to do what treatment personnel suggested:

> And when I was in a program, if I had a counselor running a group, and he ain't experienced some of the things that I experienced, I wouldn't listen to him. I would question him. "Dude, you ever been in jail?" And he would say no, so how would he tell me about jail? "You ever been in the projects?" "No." "Well, how you gonna tell me about the projects then?" And I was real stubborn like that for a while. After I been in the program for a little while, then it dawned on me that if I learn what he knows, I'll have what he knows, I'll know what I know, and I'm twice as smart.

Black described how his wife points out consequences of his behavior:

> It all comes back to my wife, she helped me see a lot of that...[she would say], "You know this jail stuff is gonna have to stop 'cause it's not going to work. I love you, you love me, but with TJ here I mean, when are you going to give it up? You say you love us, but you want to continue to you know"—So she was like, "You know sometimes the risk is just not worth it." Because I'm like, "I'm doing this for us," and she's like, "No, you're not." But that's my way of trying to justify me doing what I wanted to do, and she's like, "cause we don't want you to go to jail."

Jay said that through treatment, he learned several things: that people are not out to get him, he can trust others' guidance, and that he does not always have to be right. He learned from treatment staff that if he changed his thinking, he could change his behavior. He said, "I didn't get in the way. I just followed through with what I was told." He said he regularly checks his thinking with others before he acts.

Bama reported that he got a sponsor for the first time, works the steps, and makes and keeps AA commitments. Nick stated that he manages by doing what his MH therapist tells him and by making a commitment to be honest with her. Brother Nawapo described developing a daily structure with the help of residential staff and his MH therapist which includes taking his HIV and psychotropic medication and eating meals at set times. E said that AA gave him a set of instructions and tools that have never failed him since he has been sober. He has used those guidelines as a means to internalize new ways to function.

E said:

> For a long, long time, I blamed my mom. And this time when I got sober, my sponsor asked me if I had ever, as I was going through like my fourth step with resentments towards her, considered that maybe she was doing the best she could. And I hadn't. And that like instantly freed me of any resentment I had towards her. So we have a good relationship today.

Being Careful About Engaging in Intimate Relationships Six study respondents, Lee, E, Nick, Jay, Ace, and Brother Nawapo, discussed their decisions to carefully manage intimate relationships, describing that the additional affective demands of those relationship caused negative impacts on respondents' thought processes and behavior. Wyse, Harding and Morenoff (2008) discussed the importance to their respondents of maintaining positive intimate attachments but their simultaneous wariness of these attachments because respondents' risk of recidivism was so closely linked to intimate partners' behavior.

Jay and Ace reported that they were avoiding relationships until they felt more stable. E stated that he had just broken up with his son's mother because he was not happy and was not being honest with himself about it. He was single and said he would remain so until he decided what he wanted. Brother Nawapo reported that he broke off a relationship with a woman because she was a substance abuser. Although Nick was engaged in an intimate relationship at the time of the interview, he said he chose to remain homeless rather than live with his girlfriend for fear that living together would threaten the relationship.

Lee stated that his binges often began due to issues he was having with his intimate partners. He said that this time, he is following his sponsor's advice to "stay away from women" until he is ready. He asked rhetorically, "How you gonna love someone else if you don't love yourself first?" Lee is not sure when he will be ready but trusts that his sponsor will know.

Daily Conscious Decisions Nine respondents (Nick, Ace, Black, Brother Nawapo, Pink Panther, Mark, Dee, Jay, and Lee) discussed needing to make conscious decisions concerning self-care in order to avoid impulsive actions or behavior damaging to themselves or others. This self-management technique was shared by Haggard et al.'s (2001) respondents who described themselves as preoccupied with thoughts of identifying situations that could cause problems, such as getting into fights. These daily conscious decisions are also indicative of respondents' changes of thought process about what they need to do to avoid antisocial behavior. They then put those determinations into action.

Nick said that he had to learn to deal with things differently so that he did not make the same mistake. He said that he was writing in a journal, taking his psychotropic medication, attending therapy regularly, avoiding conflicts "at all costs," and maintaining a self-care regimen, all learned as a result of guidance provided by his MH therapist.

Ace described giving careful consideration to his housing situation. He moved away from his hometown, stating that being away from familiar areas and people helped him to avoid his old behaviors. He first lived in a shelter and then rented a room rather than moving in with family so that he could learn to be on his own and set his own goals. He reported doing volunteer work, attending church, visiting with his family regularly, and making sure to count his blessings.

Black said he made conscious decisions every day to keep quiet and utilize social avoidance strategies to avoid conflict. Jay focused on making sure that he followed through with promises. He said, "Whatever I say I'm going to do, I try my best."

Brother Nawapo said that he learned from his MH therapist to count writing his angry thoughts down as an action instead of acting on them. He reported that he was keeping to himself except at the sober house and AA meetings, also utilizing social avoidance strategies to avoid conflicts.

If he could not avoid a conflict, he reported that he would apologize for his part of it. He stated that he is "a better person and a more productive member of society," a clear identity shift, due to setting goals and boundaries to avoid violence, skills he readily attributes to his MH therapist.

Pink Panther reported that he moved away from home to be away from bad influences. At the time of the interview, he was living in a shelter while waiting for Social Security Disability and housing. He reported that he learned to be humble and that he listened a lot to others. He was attending AA meetings six times per week and taking psychotropic medication for the first time.

Mark described a very stressful work environment at the correctional halfway house where he was constantly being challenged by the residents, who he referred to as "program gangsters." He relied strongly on the support and guidance of his supervisor to avoid responding aggressively. Dee said that he did not have to make conscious decisions to avoid violence; he "is not on that level anymore." But he described carefully avoiding conflicts and said that when he was wrong, he apologized. He said, "I think twice before I act out."

A real-time example of impulse control, behavioral change, and identity change occurred during my interview with Jay. The staff person at the sober house graciously ceded the only office to me so that I could meet there with Jay. At the beginning of our meeting, he mentioned that he had found another resident's wallet earlier that day. Mid-way through the interview, the staff person (who knew Jay had the wallet) knocked on the door. She told him that the resident was about to walk back to the grocery store to see if his wallet had been left there. Jay handed it over with all of the money intact so she could return it to the resident. He described being proud of himself for being able to do that.

Societal Obstacles to Secondary Desistance

Successful desistance from the lifestyle and subculture which supports serious, long-term criminal behavior and substance abuse must involve an identity change from considering oneself a member of this marginalized community to seeing oneself as part of the larger, prosocial community. Often, people who engage in crime and chronic substance abuse were born into membership of other marginalized groups. Many are racial and ethnic minorities who were raised in poverty in urban ghettoes. Many experienced traumas as a result of this childhood including those related to community violence and family dysfunction. Resources offered to children in wealthier communities including mental health treatment and quality educational services are largely unavailable to the poor. These situations were certainly the case for many study respondents.

Furthermore, poor communities' experiences with agencies of authority can be overwhelmingly negative. Arrest and incarceration rates are higher for racial and ethnic minorities and for poor people. Abuse of authority including violent and assaultive behavior toward those under police and correctional control occurs more frequently in poor communities and in communities of color. From a very early age, children growing up in poverty can acquire a negative perception of the communities outside of their own. Therefore, the desire to engage with and become part of this larger community becomes a very difficult endeavor.

In a reciprocal manner, American society holds an intensely disparaging view of those engaged in criminal behavior. Maruna, LeBel, Mitchell and Naples (2004) described this as a "negativity bias" in which a single deviant act can stigmatize a person in perpetuity while any amount of prosocial behaviors may never alter this designation. A violent act worsens the bias. It is viewed as a dominant, stable trait that is malicious and dangerous at its essence, more deserving of punishment and more difficult to reform than other criminal acts (Hochstetler, Copes, & Williams, 2010). As this label becomes increasingly entrenched, deviance as an ongoing self-state is internalized by the offender (Goffman, 1963; Maruna, 2001). Current conservative cultural, social, and political trends reinforce the exclusion and consequent isolation of offenders and ex-offenders (Garland, 2001). These societal reactions bedevil the identification processes which produce the identity shift necessary to enable secondary desistance.

Summary

Secondary desistance involves changing self-perception, long-term patterns of functioning, habits and routines, coping strategies, personal philosophies, ideas about other people, one's sense of the larger community, and the perception of one's place in that community. Along with evolving life circumstances, personal growth and change occur in tandem with the aging process, one's own and those of one's significant others. It is a massive endeavor and one that is not a finite process.

Respondents' desistance involved a pathway which integrated their life circumstances and situations, significant relationships, and internal psychological capacities. Some respondents engaged in a two-phase path, primary and then secondary, where serious crime was first relinquished followed by the renunciation of all criminal behavior and substance abuse. Others leapt directly from a criminal lifestyle to one of a prosocial community member.

Every study participant talked about the experience of learning to change his thought processes about his dysfunctional behavior by accepting the guidance of a trusted other who often functioned as a role model. Several men discussed the positive impact of the death of a significant other who had enabled their criminal behavior and substance abuse. Many talked about the need to accept and utilize social service resources and to share emotions within a supportive community. The importance of a sense of belonging within the larger community was often experienced by raising children or being seen as a role model by younger family members.

In order for this shift to become integrated within themselves, respondents had to engage in an identity change process. In their narratives, they described it as brought about by affective, cognitive, and behavioral changes, resulting from their relationships with significant others. Through identification processes, both identifying with others and being able to identify others as like oneself, respondents internalized new thoughts and feelings and learned coping strategies. These new mental capacities produced new types of judgment, decision making, and boundary setting skills which were applied to changing their behavior. As respondents' affective and cognitive capacities strengthened and their behavior changed consistently, identity was reformulated based on these new patterns of functioning. And these new emotional, cognitive, and behavioral habits and routines serve to reinforce the internal identity shift which produced them.

Substance abuse and mental health treatment organizations are well positioned to function as a bridge between these two identities and communities. As members of the larger community, counselors and therapists represent the rejecting aspects of our culture, yet due to their training and function, their goal is one of integration and inclusion. They are best suited to promote the identificatory, affective, cognitive, and behavioral mechanisms necessary for clients to achieve and maintain long-term sobriety and prosocial behavior.

Part III of the book focuses on treatment with criminal and addicted clients. Chapter 5 explores the diagnostic complexities of the dually and triply diagnosed. Chapter 6 proposes a practice theory which demonstrates effective relationally based techniques to facilitate secondary desistance. And Chap. 7 applies relational concepts and interventions to current practice protocols.

References

Aresti, A., Eatough, V., & Brooks-Gordon, B. (2010). Doing time after time: An interpretive phenomenological analysis of reformed ex-prisoners' experiences of self change, identity and career opportunities. *Psychology, Crime & Law, 16*, 169–190.

Bahr, S. J., Harris, L., Fisher, J. K., & Armstrong, A. H. (2010). Successful reentry: What differentiates successful and unsuccessful parolees? *International Journal of Offender Therapy and Comparative Criminology, 54*, 667–692.

Byrne, C. F., & Trew, K. J. (2008). Pathways through crime: The development of crime and desistance in the accounts of men and women offenders. *The Howard Journal, 47*, 238–258.

Farrall, S. (2004). Supervision, motivation, and social context: What matters most when probationers desist. In G. Mair (Ed.), *What matters most in probation* (pp. 187–209). Cullompton, UK: Willan Publishing.

Farrall, S., & Calverley, A. (2006). *Understanding desistance from crime: Theoretical directions in resettlement and rehabilitation*. Maidenhead: Open University Press.

Garland, D. (2001). *The culture of control: Crime and social order in contemporary society*. Chicago: Chicago University Press.

Glaser, D. (1969). *The effectiveness of a prison and parole system* (Abridgedth ed.). Indianapolis, IN: Bobbs-Merrill.

Goffman, E. (1963). *Stigma: Notes on the management of spoiled identity*. Englewood Cliffs, NJ: Prentice-Hall.

Haggard, U., Gumpert, C. H., & Grann, M. (2001). Against all odds: A qualitative follow-up study of high risk violent offenders who were not reconvicted. *Journal of Interpersonal Violence, 16*, 1048–1065.

Hochstetler, A., Copes, H., & Williams, J. P. (2010). "That's not who I am": How offenders commit violent acts and reject authentically violent selves. *Justice Quarterly, 27*, 492–516.

Hughes, M. (1998). Turning points in the lives of young inner-city men forgoing destructive criminal behaviors: A qualitative study. *Social Work Research, 22*, 143–150.

Irwin, J. (1970). *The felon*. Englewood Cliffs, NJ: Prentice-Hall.

Leibrich, J. (1993). *Straight to the point: Angles on giving up crime*. Dunedin: University of Otago Press.

Maruna, S. (2001). *Making good: How ex-convicts reform and rebuild their lives*. Washington, DC: American Psychological Association.

Maruna, S., LeBel, T. P., Mitchell, N., & Naples, M. (2004). Pygmalion in the reintegration process: Desistance from crime through the looking glass. *Psychology, Crime and the Law, 10*, 271–281.

Meisenhelder, T. (1982). Becoming normal: Certification as a stage in exiting from crime. *Deviant Behavior: An Interdisciplinary Journal, 3*, 137–153.

Pithers, W. (1990). Relapse prevention with sexual aggressors: A method for maintaining therapeutic gain and enhancing external supervision. In W. L. Marshall, D. R. Laws, & H. E. Barbaree (Eds.), *Handbook of sexual assault: Issues, theories, and treatment of the offender* (pp. 343–362). New York: Plenum Press.

Presser, L. (2008). *Been a heavy life: Stories of violent men*. Urbana: University of Illinois Press.

Rains-Russell, L. (2009). *The role of felony probations' families in the desistance process* (Doctoral dissertation). Retrieved from Proquest Dissertation Abstracts International. (UMI number: 3367246).

Saldana, J. (2013). *The coding manual for qualitative researchers* (2nd ed.). Los Angeles: Sage Publications.

Sampson, R. J., & Laub, J. H. (1993). *Crime in the making: Pathways and turning points through life*. Cambridge, MA: Harvard University Press.

Sampson, R. J., & Laub, J. H. (2003). Life-course desisters? Trajectories of crime among delinquent boys followed to age 70. *Criminology, 41*, 555–592.

Walker, L. (2010). 'His mam, my dad, my girlfriend, loads of people used to bring him up': The value of social support for (ex) offender fathers. *Child & Family Social Work, 15*, 238–247.

Wyse, J., Harding, D. J., & Morenoff, J. (2008). *Romantic relationships and criminal desistance: Moving beyond marriage*. Paper presented at the American Sociological Association, Boston, MA.

Part III

Practice

The third section of the book integrates relational concepts, the analysis of respondents' narratives, and case examples to elucidate the therapy process with this client population. The complexities encountered during the diagnosis process are explored in Chap. 5. Confusion about usage of the ICD-9, ICD-10, and DSM-5 are discussed and deficiencies of the relevant diagnoses including Antisocial Personality and Substance Abuse are explored. The author proposes a practice theory in Chap. 6 which incorporates relational theory into the assessment, working phases, and termination stages of treatment. Therapeutic conflict, so commonly occurring with this client population, is highlighted. Chapter 7 applies the basic concepts of the treatment model to the real world of publicly funded agencies, time-limited Cognitive Behavioral Therapy, and group modalities.

5

Diagnostic Considerations

Abstract Diagnoses can be a useful organizing concept with which to begin treatment. However, the USA is currently experiencing a transition from sole use of the DSM-5 to the tenth editions of the ICD as a diagnostic reference. These manuals differ substantively in their respective treatments of antisocial personality disorder (ASPD) and the continuum of substance abuse disorders. There appears to be much similarity and lack of clarity between the criteria lists of these two diagnoses. Additionally, neither diagnostic manual addresses dynamic differences between ASPD and psychopathy. Treatability of these disorders is addressed. Diagnostic impressions of the respondent group are presented including additional factors of post traumatic stress disorder, major mental illness, physiological illnesses, and sociocultural factors affecting diagnosis.

The section on treatment begins with diagnosis as it is an important organizing concept. No matter the philosophy or scope of intervention, the categorization of presenting symptoms and issues is one of the preliminary steps of treatment; it establishes parameters for the treatment plan. However, many complexities plague this process particularly when assessing a client population suffering from multiple psychiatric illnesses and social vulnerabilities.

© The Editor(s) (if applicable) and The Author(s) 2016

D.H. Benveniste, *Changing Substance Abuse and Criminal Behavior Through Therapeutic Relationships*, DOI 10.1057/978-1-137-53039-4_5

Even the method of diagnosing is in a state of flux. Most countries employ the tenth edition of the International Classification of Diseases (ICD-10) published by the World Health Organization (WHO) in 1992 for purposes of diagnosis. The USA has relied upon the American Psychiatric Association's (APA) Diagnostic and Statistical Manual, now in its fifth edition (DSM-5) published in 2013. US federal regulation requires a shift to the sole usage of the ICD-10 in 2015.

This chapter will address both texts. Although they list the same illnesses, their formulations are divergent. For the purposes of this chapter, DSM-5 diagnoses are listed first, followed by the ICD-10 terminology and criteria. The diagnoses typically used in conjunction with this population include antisocial personality disorder/dissocial personality disorder (ASPD/DPD) and substance-related and addictive disorders/ mental and behavioural disorders due to psychoactive substance use.

There appears to be some leakage among the criminal behavior and substance abuse diagnoses. Psychopathy, an additional illness, is conflated with sociopathy in the diagnostic manuals yet deserves its own classification. Although criminal behaviors may connect the two, the type of crime committed and the dynamics of the offender are dissimilar. Treatability of the disorders is addressed in this chapter.

Diagnostic impressions of the respondent group are presented in order to illustrate some of the challenges and treatment implications of the diagnostic process. Post Traumatic Stress Disorder (PTSD), a diagnosis not typically utilized when assessing a client with ASPD/DPD, appears relevant in understanding the psychological issues of the respondent group. Respondents present a final diagnostic conundrum: how to diagnose those with previous histories of behavior at odds with current functioning.

Antisocial/Dissocial Personality Disorder

- A pervasive pattern of disregard for and violation of the rights of others
- Failure to conform to social norms
- Deceitfulness
- Impulsivity or failure to plan ahead
- Irritability and aggressiveness

- Reckless disregard for the safety of self and others
- Consistent irresponsibility: repeated failure to sustain consistent work or honor financial obligations
- Lack of remorse

Viewing this list outside of its context within the DSM-5 (APA, 2013), a substance abuse counselor might conclude that these primarily behavioral descriptors refer to someone with a chronic substance abuse problem as many of these traits and behaviors predominate when illegal substances are used as a primary coping mechanism. However, this list is not found in the DSM-5 section on use of substances; they are the criteria for ASPD. Increasing the ambiguity, these criteria describe severe and persistent substance abuse while also accurately describing those suffering from severe and persistent poverty.

Although societal vulnerabilities such as racial minority status and poverty are not listed in the diagnostic manuals as such, some theorists (for example, Walsh & Wu, 2008; Wilson, 2014) believe that bias toward the poor and criminal populations, both of whom are disproportionately comprised of racial minorities, is evidenced in the conceptualization of the ASPD/DPD diagnosis. Wilson (2014) stated that one of the most prominent complaints about the ASPD/DPD disorder is its predominant focus on behavioral symptoms associated with criminality rather than on any underlying psychological processes.

Walsh & Wu (2008) venture further to question whether the ASPD/DPD diagnosis should even qualify as a psychiatric disorder, stating that the diagnosis describes aspects of socio-cultural status and not mental illness. "Poverty is soul wrenching; it breeds anger, envy, hopelessness, and despair, all of which in turn lead to an elevated risk of violence, including violence against children" (p. 146). From this perspective, poverty is the cause of crime and criminal behavior is the main criterion for the diagnosis of ASPD.

The ICD-10 (WHO, 1992) approaches these areas more helpfully in terms of the task of diagnosis. In the Notes for Users section of the ICD-10 Classification of Mental and Behavioural Disorders: Diagnostic Criteria for Research (1993), authors from the World Health Organization declare the general ICD rule of avoiding the use of social role performance as a diagnostic criterion, listing DPD as an "unavoidable exception." Their description is as follows:

> Personality disorder characterized by disregard for social obligations, and callous unconcern for the feelings of others. There is gross disparity between behaviour and the prevailing social norms. Behaviour is not readily modifiable by adverse experience, including punishment. There is a low tolerance to frustration and a low threshold for discharge of aggression, including violence; there is a tendency to blame others, or to offer plausible rationalizations for the behaviour bringing the patient into conflict with society.

While the DSM-5 description reflects the influences of poverty, the ICD-10 description is more useful in formulating a treatment plan, despite also having an emphasis on antisocial behavior. It includes personality characteristics and weaknesses, indicating directions to take in treatment (low frustration tolerance and threshold for discharge of aggression) as well as traits that present obstacles to treatment (behavior not readily modifiable by adverse experience and the tendency to blame others). However, these criteria could still easily describe the traits of a chronic substance abuser.

Substance Abuse

The DSM-5 (APA, 2013) devotes 110 pages to substance-related disorders delineating ten classes of drugs (and one category describing problem gambling). These disorders are further demarcated into two groups, substance use (SU) and substance-induced disorders, such as intoxication and withdrawal. The chapter is organized by substance; clinicians are instructed to list each substance as a separate diagnosis rather than diagnosing by characteristics of the user.

Under each substance group, alcohol, cannabis, hallucinogens, inhalants, opioid substances, sedatives, stimulants, and tobacco, is found a list of the same criteria to determine the diagnosis. The list includes: a problematic pattern of use leading to significant impairment or distress; the substance is often taken in larger amounts or over a longer period than was intended; a desire to reduce or control use; a great deal of time is spent in activities necessary to obtain the substance or recover from its effects; craving; failure to fulfill major role obligations at work, home, or school; continued use despite social or interpersonal problems; important social, occupational, or recreational activities are given up or reduced because of the substance; recurrent use when it is physically hazardous; use is continued despite knowledge of having a problem with it; tolerance to the substance; and withdrawal when attempting to stop (APA, 2013).

Outside of the criteria specific to use of the substance (for example, desire to reduce or control use, tolerance, and withdrawal), the list of diagnostic criteria for the substance groups is very similar to that of ASPD. The main difference between them is the negative valence of the ASPD terminology. Both sets of diagnoses address the lack of responsibility in carrying out life tasks, danger to self or other, and the interpersonal problems that result from having the diagnosis but the ASPD criterion includes language such as "consistent irresponsibility," "repeated failure to sustain consistent work or honor financial obligations," "reckless disregard for the safety of self and others," and "a pervasive pattern of disregard for and violation of the rights of others" (APA, 2013).

The language of the SU criteria is more neutral: "failure to fulfill major responsibilities," "recurrent use where it is physically hazardous," and "continued use despite persistent or recurrent social or interpersonal problems" (APA, 2013). The emotional or interpersonal criteria listed in the ASPD diagnosis, irritability, deceitfulness, impulsivity, aggressiveness, and lack of remorse, often apply to substance abusers but are not included in that section.

There are two criteria of ASPD that do not appear in the description of SU. The first is failure to conform to social norms, which does apply to some substance users, and most certainly to the respondents of this study. Age of onset is specified for ASPD, beginning at age 18 with a history of conduct disorder prior to age 15. The SU diagnosis does not specify age of onset but indicates that adults age 18–24 have a relatively high prevalence of substance usage (APA, 2013).

The ICD-10's (WHO, 1992) treatment of substance abuse is also different from the DSM-5. Firstly, this section is called "Mental and Behavioural Disorders Due to Psychoactive Substance Use" and not

"Substance Related and Addictive Disorders," maintaining the focus on people rather than substances. The descriptors of use are grouped under: acute intoxication, harmful use, dependence syndrome, withdrawal state, withdrawal state with delirium, psychotic disorder, amnesic syndrome, and residual and late-onset psychotic disorder. The dependence syndrome corresponds closely to the SU DSM-5 criteria. These categories provide more depth and breadth about the nature of the substance use than the DSM-5's method of employing the same criteria for all types of use. However, diagnostic questions remain that neither manual addresses.

Neither the DSM-5 nor the ICD-10 provides guidance about how to distinguish chronic substance abuse from antisocial personality. Neither manual lists substance use, abuse, or dependence as a criterion of ASPD/DPD yet substance abuse commonly co-occurs in those diagnosed with the personality disorders. Wilson (2014) stated that up to 90% of those diagnosed with ASPD also abuse substances. Criminal activity is often necessary to obtain funds to maintain an addiction to illegal substances. The functional difference between these two diagnoses occurring simultaneously, or being co-morbid, as opposed to the diagnoses sharing their criteria, is unclear.

In the case of severe and persistent SU, it is also unclear whether or not the ASPD/DPD diagnosis applies. Someone who is addicted to opioids, crack cocaine, or methamphetamine, for example, will meet the criteria for the personality disorders that include disregard of others and social norms. The difference between the two becomes visible when the abuse stops. Recovering drug addicts with antisocial tendencies will continue to violate the law. Those without the personality disorder will not.

Alcohol and cannabis use present more complex diagnostic issues. The easy and legal access to alcohol most often eliminates ASPD/DPD criteria which apply to illegal use. And because the effects of alcohol and cannabis are largely determined by the amount consumed, compared to heroin or crack cocaine for example, a fixed set of criteria for dependence is inadequate to diagnose the type of use.

Although both manuals permit coding for severity, it is defined by the number of criteria met and not the seriousness of each criterion. For example, the DSM-5's (APA, 2013) first criterion, "a problematic pattern of use leading to significant impairment or distress," does not define the term "significant." The manuals lack a diagnostic continuum of dependence indicating a range of severity which would permit clinicians to distinguish functional users from the more severely addicted. Additionally, the severe end of the abuse continuum should include some of the descriptors from the ASPD criteria list including: deceitfulness, irritability, impulsivity, lack of remorse, and reckless disregard for the safety of themselves and others.

Lastly, chronic substance abuse of any type involves the reliance on a substance to moderate affect, reduce anxiety, and disinhibit self-control. Long-term use of an external support would indicate chronic weakness or deficit in the personality structure. However, Flores (2004) distinguished three possible diagnostic scenarios concerning the interrelation between personality disorders and substance abuse. He stated that it is impossible to determine until the person is sober whether (1) substance abuse is a symptom of an existing personality disorder, (2) chemically dependent people are manifesting symptoms of a personality disorder due to the effects of the substances in their systems, or (3) there is a common factor that produces both disorders. He said, "The stress and regressive pull that prolonged substance use has on the brain and the body often blurs the distinction between the two disorders" (p. 29). Neither manual provides adequate guidance about how or when to differentiate chronic use from personality disorders or how to understand the interaction between the diagnoses.

ASPD/DPD and Psychopathy

ASPD/DPD is also known as sociopathy and those who suffer from it as sociopaths. While the term "psychopathy" referring to psychopaths is conflated with ASPD/DPD in the DSM-5 and ICD-10, psychopaths differ from sociopaths in important ways. Meloy (1988) defined psychopathy as a "deviant developmental disturbance characterized by an inordinate amount of instinctual aggression and the absence of an object relational capacity to bond" (p. 5). The defining characteristic of psychopathy is the brain's lack of ability to connect cognitive and emotional networks. This discontinuity causes severe emotional deficits and a lack of an emotional basis for self-regulation (Walsh & Wu, 2008).

According to Walsh and Wu (2008), psychopathy is biological in origin and its prevalence remains fairly stable across cultures, social classes, and time periods. Occurrence of psychopathy in the general US population falls between 1% and 3% of males and less than 1% of females (Pemmet, 2013; Walsh & Wu, 2008). Factor analysis of the PCL-R, the Psychopathy Checklist-Revised developed by Robert Hare (1996), indicated that 15–25% of offenders diagnosed with ASPD meet PCL-R criteria for psychopathy (Walsh & Wu, 2008). This result demonstrates that the vast majority of offenders diagnosed with ASPD (75–85%) do not meet the PCL-R criteria for psychopathy. It is therefore possible to view psychopathy as a subset of ASPD. To clarify, all psychopaths meet the criteria for ASPD but relatively few sociopaths meet the criteria for psychopathy.

Although sociopaths and psychopaths share aggression as a common trait, Meloy (1988) distinguished affective aggression from psychopathic predatory aggression. Affective aggression is comprised of 11 features including intense central nervous system arousal; a subjective experience of conscious emotion; a perceived threat; the goal of threat reduction; public displays of aggression-based posturing (for example, demeaning gestures or language); and a reactive violent response (if present). This type of aggression is time limited in nature and may be displaced to others present. A temporary loss of self and object differentiation occurs as well as possible temporary loss of reality testing. An example is the aggressors in a barroom brawl or during an episode of road rage.

Conversely, the features of predatory aggression include minimal or absent nervous system arousal; no conscious experience of emotion; planned and purposeful violence, if present; no perceived threat; intrapsychic goals such as gratification of drives or fantasies; no displacement to others present; use of private rituals; the aggression is expressed through intentional behavior; a heightened and focused sensory awareness; and no loss of reality testing. An example is the serial rapist.

Sociopaths experience affective and not predatory aggression (Meloy, 1988). Their occurrence in the general population fluctuates with environmental and economic conditions, emanating from the lower social classes, dysfunctional families, and disadvantaged minority groups (Walsh & Wu, 2008). Pemmet (2013) further differentiated sociopathy from psychopathy based on the relative presence or absence of morality. He described psychopaths as lacking morality entirely while sociopaths have a moral code but it is at odds with that of the prevailing culture. Walsh and Wu (2008) stated that "sociopaths develop the kind of emotional calluses that psychopaths are apparently born with primarily through inadequate socialization and hostile childhood experiences" (p. 143).

Their patterns of substance use or abuse are also divergent. Meloy (1988) found a correlation between psychopathy and the use of psychostimulants such as cocaine, amphetamine, or methamphetamine. He stated that these drugs' effects compensate for the psychopath's lack of nervous system response and help to satisfy his or her need for thrill seeking. In contrast, many sociopaths use central nervous system depressants such as opiates and alcohol in order to blunt emotional pain. Much antisocial behavior that co-occurs with use of illegal substances stems from the need to support a drug habit. Those psychopaths who engage in criminal behavior do so for pleasure-seeking purposes.

To conflate sociopathy with psychopathy is to group criminal behaviors together while ignoring the physiological and psychological dynamics which produce them. Gang membership, a career of theft, and a history of substance abuse-related assaults are all consistent with sociopathy. Serial murder, serial rape, contract killing, and torture of victims indicate psychopathy. The motivations and goals of these sets of behaviors are very different and affect treatability.

Treatability

Few theorists who have studied treatment outcomes for clients who carry the ASPD/DPD and substance use disorder diagnoses have concluded that they respond well to mental health or substance abuse intervention (Dumaine, 2003; Fletcher, Nutton, & Brend, 2015; Hubbard, Craddock, & Anderson, 2003; Wilson, 2014). According to a meta-analysis by Windsor, Jemal and Alessi (2015), Cognitive Behavioral Therapy (CBT) was found to be ineffective in reducing substance abuse for African American or Hispanic clients. Poverty, often co-occurring with both criminal and substance abuse behavior, is also considered to be a confounding factor in diagnosis and treatment (Altman, 2005). Traits of deceitfulness, impulsivity, behavior dangerous to self and other, lack of concern for the feelings of others, and the chaotic and crisis-prone lifestyle of chronic poverty place inordinate demands on the treatment endeavor (Wilson, 2014). Due to these demands, clients presenting with these diagnoses are dreaded by most clinicians (Benveniste, 2012). Dumaine (2003) refers to treatment with them as "mission impossible" (p. 144).

For the purposes of relationally based therapy, the critical factor in determining treatability is the capacity to establish an emotional bond with others. Because the DSM-5 (APA, 2013) and ICD-10 (WHO, 1992) diagnostic categories in question are behaviorally defined, they do not produce guidance about this critical aspect of the treatment. Diagnoses of ASPD/DPD and/or substance abuse do not preclude the potential for clients to make effective use of relationally based therapy. The criteria only serve as a preliminary warning that the therapeutic work ahead will be complex and demanding. However, in order to distinguish the capacity to engage in a therapeutic relationship, sociopaths must be distinguished from psychopaths.

Since psychopaths cannot utilize affect to establish or maintain interpersonal relationships (Meloy, 1988), they are not treatable through relational modes of psychotherapy. Sociopaths, whose criminal behavior is based on socio-cultural pressures and not on needs to gratify sadistic fantasies, are capable of employing relationships to change their personality structure and behavior. Conflating sociopathy and psychopathy, as in the current definitions of ASPD/DPD, eliminates this important method of determining treatment suitability. Fortunately, based on Hare's (1996) study, it would appear that psychopathy occurs relatively infrequently among those diagnosed with ASPD/DPD.

Diagnostic Impressions of the Respondent Group

The research interview process did not include a formal diagnostic assessment as doing so would have been contrary to the purposes of the study. The goals of this book also preclude a focus on full diagnostic assessments. The intention of this section is to highlight difficulties and challenges in the process of diagnosing clients such as my respondent group, those suffering from multiple diagnoses, severe societal vulnerabilities, and substantial disabilities. Significant information relevant to the diagnosis process was shared by respondents. They discussed their backgrounds, traumatic environments and events, symptoms, substance abuse, use of SA and MH treatment, and methods of maintaining sobriety and prosocial behavior, providing enough information for me to suggest preliminary diagnostic impressions.

Sociopathy

The ASPD/DPD categorizations are functionally useless for diagnosing the respondent group for two reasons. Because the criteria are behaviorally based and all respondents engaged in the behavior, it does not allow for distinguishing among them as individuals. Additionally, all respondents reported being crime-free for as long as they had been sober. Therefore, they would not have met the criteria for ASPD/DPD at the time of the interview. ASPD/DPD would not apply because the diagnoses require current symptomatology (APA, 2013). Given respondents' histories, it would be important to be able to code for a history of ASPD/DPD but the language of the diagnostic manuals does not permit it.

For the purposes of this section, I am proposing a brief, altered version of the ASPD/DPD diagnosis. It is comprised of psychological and psychodynamic concepts more helpful in determining internal characterological structure and treatment formulations. I will apply these criteria to what respondents shared about their past behavior.

- Thought process which rejects prevailing societal norms and rules
- Low tolerance of affective states
- Primary use of external means to achieve emotional stability, for example, substances, aggressive behavior, or criminal behavior
- Perceives others as a means of achieving their own ends, sense of entitlement, hostile dependence
- Lack of ability to perceive risks to safety for self or others

Using this description of sociopathy, 6 of 11 respondents met the criteria prior to desistance: E, Mark, Brother Nowapo, Ace, Jay, and Black.

Each internalized a moral code which did not match that of the larger society, permitting rule breaking, criminal behavior, and an "us versus them" mentality. People were used to achieving their own ends, for example, Brother Nowapo robbing the drug dealers whom he was supposed to look out for and Jay and Black expecting their mothers to support them during their incarcerations. All relied on substances and criminal behavior to manage their affective states and all engaged in dangerous behavior while being blind to its risks.

Lee, Bama, Dee, Pink Panther, and Nick did not meet this set of criteria for sociopathy. Although they all had low tolerance for affective states and used external means to achieve emotional stability, the criminal thought process and relational deficits were not present. Lee and Bama used substances to opt out of the demands of adult life. Both spent their time escaping through alcohol. Bama tended to lead a solitary existence while Lee attempted relationships but would become aggressive when the interpersonal demands superseded his abilities. Dee and Pink Panther were employed for most of the time they used substances. Their moral code seemed to be in accordance with that of the larger community. Nick only committed one crime and reported that he did not abuse substances. Despite relying on others a great deal, he was mindful of the impact when he asked for help and tried to minimize his requests.

Substance Use/Dependence Syndrome

All of the respondents except for Nick reported that they had engaged in long-term, severe, and chronic substance abuse. Bama's substance of choice was alcohol. The remainder of the group were polysubstance-dependent, using a combination of marijuana, heroin, cocaine/crack cocaine, alcohol, and tobacco. However, seven of the group, E, Mark, Ace, Jay, Black, Ace, and Brother Nowapo, reported having been sober for 3 years or more. They would not carry an SU diagnosis. Bama and Dee reported about 1 year of sobriety while Pink Panther and Lee had been sober for less than 6 months. It would be possible in these cases to indicate a history of SU.

Psychopathy

Since there is no psychopathy diagnosis present in either manual, it would not be possible to assess the presence of psychopathic traits using the DSM-5 or ICD-10. Using Meloy's (1988) descriptors of predatory aggression as diagnostic criteria, it appeared to me that two of the respondents, E and Brother Nowapo, showed psychopathic traits.

E's description of his lifelong fascination with violence sounded as if it might be psychopathic in nature. Even after many years of maintaining sobriety and abstaining from criminal behavior, he talked about enjoying concerts with "mosh pits" where he would assault his compatriots with impunity and then want to give them a hug after the song was over. For him, there was no functional difference between the physical contact of an assault versus a hug. Additionally, he described himself as a "professional client" which indicates a lack of ability to engage emotionally in treatment.

However, E stated that the reason he gave up violent criminal behavior was due to his relationship with his father and he adored his infant son. His drug of choice was heroin, a narcotic used to modulate emotional pain. Therefore, it would appear that E developed some psychopathic traits perhaps in response to his horrific childhood abuse but that his overall character was capable of establishing and maintaining relationships.

When Brother Nowapo recounted assaulting people in his past, he appeared delighted in the telling. He would laugh in a merry way, relishing the memories, and not manifesting any indicators of shame or embarrassment. At the time of the interview, Brother Nowapo reported that he continued to struggle with avoiding aggressive responses. Because of the fragility of his coping skills, he would employ social avoidance strategies and isolate himself from others. It seemed that this was a difficult method for Brother Nowapo as he clearly enjoyed interacting with people.

However, Brother Nowapo described affectively -based aggression. He was angry at the people he assaulted. He also described attachments to treatment personnel, the program director at his residential program and his MH therapist, which motivated him to improve his behavior. And he expressed guilt and remorse about his violent behavior. Additionally, due to Brother Nowapo's brutal childhood and several other factors discussed below which impact his functioning, it would seem that he did not meet the criteria for a full diagnosis of psychopathy. All of the other respondents described affective aggression, acting in response to a perceived threat, which indicated sociopathy rather than psychopathy.

The presence of psychopathic traits should be carefully evaluated in order to assess their impact on treatability. In both of these cases, each respondent's psychopathic traits were balanced with indicators of a capacity to engage emotionally with others. However, the presence and severity of psychopathic traits is inversely proportional to the ability to utilize relationally based treatment.

Post Traumatic Stress Disorder

The role of environmental trauma in many respondents' lives put them at risk for Post Traumatic Stress Disorder (PTSD). The DSM-5 (APA, 2013) diagnostic criteria for PTSD include exposure to actual or physical threat of death, serious injury, or sexual violence; distressing dreams or memories associated with the event; dissociative reactions in which it feels as if the trauma were recurring; prolonged distress at cues which represent the event; persistent avoidance of stimuli which represent the event; lack of ability to remember aspects of the event; negative belief system; persistent negative emotional state; inability to experience positive emotions; feelings of detachment from others; irritability or angry outbursts; reckless or self-destructive behavior; hypervigilance; and sleep disturbance.

The ICD-10's (WHO, 1992) diagnostic criteria are mostly the same as those of the DSM-5 other than the first criterion, the source of the disorder. The ICD-10 includes physical injury or severe mental or emotional distress, such as military combat, violent assault, natural disaster, or having cancer as events with the potential to produce PTSD. Hence, the ICD-10's sources for developing PTSD are far more wide-reaching than that of the DSM-5 which limits the event as exposing the person to actual or physical threat of death.

It is interesting to note the intersections of PTSD, ASPD/DPD, and SU, particularly irritability and angry outbursts and reckless or self-destructive behavior. If chronic environmental stressors such as poverty or life in a dangerous ghetto were included in the sources for PTSD, it would be possible to conclude that some of the symptoms ascribed to ASPD/DPD actually derive from PTSD. PTSD and substance abuse also have a high rate of co-occurrence (Brown, Stout, & Gannon-Rowley, 1998). However, as opposed to ASPD/DPD and substance abuse disorders, PTSD is considered to be treatable through several psychotherapeutic interventions including talk therapy, EMDR, medication, and psychoeducation. (See Foa, Keane, & Friedman, 2009 for a comprehensive discussion of PTSD treatment methods.)

Based on their narratives, seven of the respondents, Mark, Brother Nowapo, Dee, Nick, E, Black, and Pink Panther, described events which met the criteria for the source of PTSD. Mark was sexually assaulted as a child and physically abused by his mother. Brother Nowapo witnessed the murder of his father as a child. Dee was beaten regularly by his brother. Nick was sexually assaulted by his brother as a child and in prison when he was in late teens. E described horrific abuse at the hands of his mother. Black discussed being the victim of violence in his neighborhood when young. Pink Panther watched his girlfriend die from cancer. If chronic environmental stressors were included as a source of PTSD, the remainder of the group, Lee, Bama, Ace, and Jay, could also be included as meeting the first criterion of PTSD.

However, experiencing an event which could trigger PTSD does not necessarily cause the disorder. In order for the diagnosis to apply, a majority of the other criteria must be met including the intrusive and avoidant symptoms as well as the alterations of cognitions and mood. It could be that the heavy use of substances by most respondents was an attempt at self-medication to lessen the symptoms of PTSD. Since aggressive behavior can be understood as a response to a sense of chronic threat, and negative emotion, anger, and irritability are included in the PTSD symptom list, it is possible to view respondents' behavior as PTSD-based symptomatology as much as it was an indicator of ASPD/DPD.

The role of dissociation in trauma, so central to the relational analytical theory's model of the mind, plays a relatively minor role in PTSD criteria. Researchers are somewhat unclear about the relationship between dissociation and the development of PTSD. (For example, see Briere, Scott, & Weathers, 2005.) The DSM-5 (APA, 2013) and ICD-10 (WHO, 1992) each maintain a section of dissociative disorders (for example, Dissociative Identity Disorder and Depersonalization/Derealization Disorder) separate from the stress-based disorders.

This bifurcation of categories can cause confusion when attempting to gauge dissociative symptomatology in clients who suffer from PTSD. It also reduces the usefulness of the diagnostic categories when approaching treatment of clients from a relational stance. Although most clients would not meet the criteria for the dissociative disorders, these aspects of functioning are a main focus of relational assessment and treatment.

Major Mental Illness

Nick, Brother Nowapo, and Pink Panther reported that they had also been diagnosed with a major mental illness (schizophrenia or major or bipolar depression). Nick and Brother Nowapo said that they were receiving Social Security Disability benefits for their mental illness, and Pink Panther described being in the process of applying at the time of the interview. All three reported being prescribed multiple psychotropic medications. I did not ask about their specific diagnoses or medications. These respondents volunteered the information about their diagnoses and treatment. I was not able to determine if other respondents met the criteria for major mental illness as this assessment would have been outside of the interview parameters.

Physiological Factors Affecting Mental Functioning

Four respondents were HIV+, Brother Nowapo, Dee, Lee, and Jay. Brother Nowapo and Dee described not finding out about their disease until they began suffering symptoms. Brother Nowapo, Lee, and Jay were medication-compliant at the time of the interview. Dee reported that his doctors were not sure if he needed medication. Although his viral load was quite high, his T-cell count was also high, indicating that his system was fighting the disease. Dee was also very ambivalent about taking medication. My knowledge of the effects of HIV disease is inadequate to understand its physiological effects on mental functioning. However, its emotional impact is staggering. Lee was the only one of the group to minimize the impact of his HIV status on him perhaps because he had been diagnosed many years before and had never experienced acute symptoms.

Four respondents, Ace, Lee, Brother Nowapo, and Bama, had additional physiological conditions that impeded their cognitive abilities. Ace had diabetes which had gone untreated while he was using drugs. Lee and Bama both appeared to be suffering some brain damage from their years of heavy alcohol use. They had difficulty articulating their thoughts and remembering events. Brother Nowapo reported that he had suffered two strokes and was also diabetic. It is unknown what physiological effects the other respondents suffered from their years of substance use.

Applying for Treatment

It would appear likely that prior to their desistance from crime and substance abuse, when members of the respondent group applied for treatment, they would be diagnosed as antisocial and substance abusers. These diagnoses would not provide much guidance about the severity of their conditions or the most effective forms of treatment. It is possible that the other illnesses from which they suffered including PTSD and major mental illness would not have been considered given the high visibility of the first two. However, Brown, Stout and Gannon-Rowley (1998) stated that the majority of substance abusers interviewed for their study were not referred for PTSD treatment even when diagnosed.

With a history of longstanding desistance in place, respondents applying for treatment would look very different from their former selves. The ASPD/DPD and SU diagnoses would no longer apply. At this point, the other illnesses and physical conditions might become more evident. However, without knowing their diagnostic history, the respondents as a group would appear as if their past behaviors and pathology did not exist. In this case, the absence of the diagnoses eliminates the clinician's ability to assess client strengths.

This may appear to be a case of diagnostic quibbling as the psychosocial assessment completed at intake serves as the source of this information. However, other factors collude to reduce the efficacy of an intake interview with this client population. Poor and traumatized clients with a substantial criminal history may be suspicious of the intake process and may lie or withhold important information. Those with less education may not be as articulate about their internal states. Documentation of previous treatment attempts may not be available.

Racial minority status and poverty can have a drastic effect on treatment efficacy (Altman, 2005; Windsor, Jemal, & Alessi, 2015). Although the philosophy and intervention principles of generalist social work are organized in terms of ethnic and other minority groups and the societal and cultural problems they face, traditional mental health fields organize their interventions based on diagnoses and psychological symptoms. Given the difficulties inherent in the diagnosis process, it is illogical to dichotomize social status and mental health in this manner particularly when treating a population whose difficulties are firmly rooted in both spheres.

Due to the deficits of the ASPD/DPD and Substance Related and Addictive Disorders/Mental and Behavioural Disorders Due to Psychoactive Substance Use diagnoses, a diagnostic assessment of those suffering from these disorders will not provide guidance about treatment, particularly relationally based therapy. Furthermore, research generally confirms the intractability of these two conditions. Thus, the typical diagnostic assessment for clients with these illnesses does not provide a promising start.

Relational Diagnosis

Because the treatment model presented here is based on relational analytic theory, at the intake assessment, the clinician would need to focus on the capacity of the client to engage emotionally in relationships including the following: (1) the effects of the client's important relationships; (2) the role relationships played in facilitating both antisocial and prosocial behaviors; (3) how the client understood his or her experiences in those relationships; (4) the relational capacities the client articulated; (5) if the client reported a treatment history, an examination of his or her experiences in engaging with therapists; (6) was the therapist helpful or unhelpful and in what ways; and (7) some initial impressions of the relational capacity of the client based on his or her engagement with the intake therapist.

These aspects of psychological functioning could be ascertained during the use of pre-existing intake assessment tools. Marginalized and societally vulnerable clients would most likely present for treatment at agencies that have rigid intake procedures and clinicians would not be permitted to vary from the protocol. Therefore, it would be important to listen for these factors as an underlying theme during the intake process. However, it is often the case that the intake clinician is not the treating clinician. In this case, treating clinicians would have the information obtained during the intake process at their disposal when they first meet their new client. It would be at this point that the relational factors could be assessed.

The most important task of the intake process in terms of relationally based treatment is not to establish a diagnosis but to establish the therapy relationship, even if the clinician is going to change. The intake therapist is the first representative of the agency that the client meets face to face. The client's experiences during the course of this interview will determine his or her expectations about the potential helpfulness of the remainder of treatment. The intake interview is also the first entry for the therapist into the client's inner world.

Client presentation, including what is shared and discussed; attitude toward the therapist; demands made of the therapist, for example, for concrete services; the level of crisis the client is experiencing; and how the demands of the intake process are handled, permits the therapist to view the world from the client's point of view, including, and most importantly for relationally based treatment, how the client experiences the therapist. The therapist can formulate some initial hypotheses about the client's early experiences and significant relationships by how he or she approaches the therapist and interacts during the stressful intake process (Altman, 2005).

This narrow focus may sound reductionistic given the comprehensive requirements of the intake process. However, considering that one of the many difficulties in treating this population is its tendency to miss appointments or drop out entirely (Dumaine, 2003), establishing a warm, caring, and accepting experience for the client at intake will greatly improve the chances that he or she will follow through. As clients feel more comfortable, they generally become more willing to share accurate historical and diagnostic information about themselves.

Genuine concern, warmth, and caring by significant others were also among the most important factors study respondents credited to their transition to desistance. Clients remember when treatment staff is kind to them, particularly when they are in crisis (Padgett & Henwood, 2012). Furthermore, clients can experience kind treatment as an indication that the therapist sees something good in them. Any emotional connection such as this forged with a client, even if the treatment episode is short-lived, may begin or reinforce a desistance process.

Emphasizing the relational tasks of the intake procedure with this challenging population could provide the clinician with a new way to view the beginning of the treatment process: as more promising and hopeful than the diagnostic manuals, researchers, and many practitioners would lead us to believe. And if clinicians feel hopeful about the treatment endeavor, it will translate to clients feeling more hopeful and optimistic about the tasks they are about to face (Bromberg, 1998).

References

Altman, N. (2005). Psychoanalysis and the urban poor. In L. Aron & A. Harris (Eds.), *Relational psychoanalysis: Volume 2 innovation and expansion*. Hillsdale, NJ: Analytic Press.

American Psychiatric Association. (2013). *Diagnostic and statistical manual of mental disorders* (5th ed.). Washington, DC/London: Author.

Benveniste, D. (2012). Relational quandaries in the treatment of forensic clients. *Clinical Social Work Journal, 40*, 326–336.

Briere, J., Scott, C., & Weathers, F. (2005). Peritraumatic and persistent dissociation in the presumed etiology of PTSD. *American Journal of Psychiatry, 162*, 2295–2301.

Bromberg, P. M. (1998). *Standing in the spaces: Essays on clinical process, trauma, & dissociation*. Hillsdale, NJ/London: Analytic Press.

Brown, P. J., Stout, R. L., & Gannon-Rowley, J. (1998). Substance use disorder-PTSD comorbidity: Patients' perception of symptom interplay and treatment issues. *Journal of Substance Abuse Treatment, 15*, 445–448.

Dumaine, M. L. (2003). Meta-analysis of interventions with co-occurring disorders of severe mental illness and substance: Implications for social work practice. *Research on Social Work Practice, 13*, 142–165.

Fletcher, K., Nutton, J., & Brend, D. (2015). Attachment, a matter of substance: The potential of attachment theory in the treatment of addictions. *Clinical Social Work Journal, 43*, 109–117.

Flores, P. J. (2004). *Addiction as an attachment disorder*. Lanham, MD: Jason Aronson.

Foa, E. B., Keane, T. M., & Friedman, M. J. (Eds.). (2009). *Effective treatments for PTSD: Practice guidelines from the International Society for Traumatic Stress Studies* (2nd ed.). New York: The Guilford Press.

Hare, R. (1996). Psychopathy and antisocial personality disorder: A case of diagnostic confusion. *Psychiatric Times, 13*, 1–8.

Hubbard, R. L., Craddock, S. G., & Anderson, J. (2003). Overview of 5-year followup outcomes in the drug abuse treatment outcome studies (DATOS). *Journal of Substance Abuse Treatment, 25*, 125–134.

Meloy, J. R. (1988). *The psychopathic mind: Origins, dynamics, and treatment*. Northvale, NJ: Jason Aronson.

Padgett, D. K., & Henwood, B. F. (2012). Qualitative research for and in practice: Findings from studies with homeless adults who have serious mental illness and co-occurring substance abuse. *Clinical Social Work Journal, 40*, 187–193.

Pemmet, J. (2013). Psychopathy versus sociopathy: Why the distinction has become crucial. *Aggression and Violent Behavior, 18*, 458–461.

Walsh, A., & Wu, H. (2008). Differentiating antisocial personality disorder, psychopathy, and sociopathy: Evolutionary, genetic, neurological, and sociological considerations. *Criminal Justice Studies, 21*, 135–152.

Wilson, H. A. (2014). Can antisocial personality disorder be treated? A meta-analysis examining the effectiveness of treatment in reducing recidivism for individuals diagnosed with ASPD. *International Journal of Forensic Mental Health, 13*, 36–46.

Windsor, L. C., Jemal, A., & Alessi, E. J. (2015). Cognitive behavioral therapy: A meta-analysis of race and substance abuse outcomes. *Cultural Diversity and Ethnic Minority Psychology, 21*, 300–313.

World Health Organization. (1992). *The ICD-10 classification of mental and behavioural disorders*. Geneva: Author.

World Health Organization. (1993). *The ICD-10 classification of mental and behavioural disorders: Diagnostic criteria for research*. Geneva: Author.

6

Developing a Practice Theory

Abstract A practice theory to treat clients engaging in substance abuse and criminal behavior using the therapeutic relationship as the main mechanism of change is proposed and detailed in this chapter. Excerpts from study respondents' narratives and case examples from the author's practice are used to illustrate concepts and processes. Components of the practice theory include relationally based treatment goals; attachment-based processes, including establishing the treatment relationship, therapeutic engagement, witnessing, containment, holding, and identification; therapeutic conflict including impasses, ruptures, and enactments; resolution of enactments; the development of the capacity for internal conflict including issues related to guidance, confrontation, collusion, and enabling; the development of personal agency; identity change and moral development; and meaning making including the use of a self-narrative to promote identity cohesion.

The function of a practice or clinical theory is to transform theoretical abstractions into a useable form for therapy practice. This chapter integrates study respondents' narratives and case examples with relational psychodynamic principles to produce a practice theory for treating criminal

© The Editor(s) (if applicable) and The Author(s) 2016
D. H. Benveniste, *Changing Substance Abuse and Criminal Behavior Through Therapeutic Relationships*, DOI 10.1057/978-1-137-53039-4_6

and substance abusing clients. The framework incorporates multiple aspects of the mind that converge to produce behavior including social and interpersonal elements of family, social status, neighborhood, and culture relevant to psychological functioning and the process of treatment.

Relational goals are first presented. The major mechanisms and operations of relational therapy, attachment, identification, therapeutic conflict, personal agency, identity change, and meaning making, are each explored. Their working definitions and their function in the therapy process are examined. Results for the client, the therapist, and the therapeutic dyad are discussed. Study participants' responses relevant to these areas and clinical case examples from the author's work are incorporated into each section.

In successful relational therapy of clients with substance abuse and offending behavior, establishing, maintaining and working through issues related to attachment and therapeutic conflict are constants throughout the course of treatment. Therapeutic functions associated with establishing attachment and identification processes occur during the beginning stages of treatment and correspond with primary desistance, where some criminal behavior and substance abuse are relinquished. Capacities for internal conflict and personal agency develop during the middle stages. The end stages of treatment correlate with secondary desistance and include a complete stop to illegal and addictive behavior. Identity formation and change is addressed here. Lastly, meaning making integrates all of the previous processes and goals into an internalized system that solidifies changes.

Relationally Based Practice Theory Goals

To establish parameters for the practice theory, first it is helpful to establish relationally based treatment goals. The goal of treatment of substance abusers and offenders would appear self-evident: to avoid recidivism of the proscribed behaviors. However, rifts over goals within the substance abuse field have recently occurred. Standard CBT therapy of substance abuse based on the medical model mandates abstinence as its goal. 12 Step philosophy also espouses complete sobriety. A new treatment model, harm reduction, utilizes a public health perspective; that is to reduce but not necessarily eliminate substance use (Rothschild, 2010). On the other hand, there is no doubt about treatment goals for offenders. Complete lack of recidivism, no further criminal behavior of any type, is its intent.

The harm reduction approach is appropriate to consider with clients who are generally functional and whose substance abuse is not severe. However, it is not realistic to apply this goal to clients having problems similar to those of the study respondents. They suffer from dual and triple diagnoses and committed very serious offenses. Their drug and alcohol abuse spanned the range of DSM-5 (APA, 2013) categories of substances. Therefore, a typical treatment goal for this client population is the relinquishment of all criminal and substance abusing behaviors.

Common sense would dictate that any intervention program with these populations have abstinence as its ultimate goal. But a therapy goal must also address other areas of psychological functioning that have a direct impact on behavior: thoughts, feelings, relational capacities, social and cultural impacts, and psychological defense systems. For these purposes, it must also address the process of therapy. As this level of complexity is approached, the concept of a specific behaviorally based therapy goal becomes less easily defined.

The term "goal" assumes an end point to a linear process. However, the progression of therapy is not linear. Conditions are stabilized; symptomatology is reduced. As therapeutic work continues, the process of exploration involves circling back to understand conditions and symptoms from deeper perspectives. Regression occurs. Enactments occur. Personality structures change. Capacity improves. The therapeutic relationship is restabilized in a stronger form. More exploration occurs. More progress results.

The process is commonly compared to the peeling of the layers of an onion. To the untrained eye, the layers appear no different from each other even though each is substantially closer to the nucleus of the issues. To the client, as each level of understanding and resolution is attained, the process seems finite, only to further reveal what appear to be the same issues and problems all over again. A common refrain is, "But I know this already. Why are we here again?" They are the same and yet different; a slowly and consistently progressing feedback loop.

Secondary desistance, like sobriety, is a long-term process that never fully "arrives." Clients must continue to actively observe and monitor their self-states and behavior to avoid or manage stressors or the potential for relapse increases. 12 Step programs refer to those who do not work to maintain their recovery and are thereby at higher risk to return to substance abuse as "complacent." Successful avoidance of these behaviors entails a lifelong commitment.

Hence, relationally based goals for these client populations cannot have the same characteristics as concrete and observable behaviorally based goals. Relational goals both define and determine the processes of treatment. Each redefinition redetermines treatment processes and goals. They form an interdependent and mutually determined feedback loop of affective attunement whose goal is to reach emotional truth (Holmes, 2011). And given the co-created nature of the relationally based therapeutic relationship, goals must also be co-created.

This practice theory proposes a dual set of goals to begin the therapy: one for the therapist and one for the client. Beginning with those applying to any relationally based treatment, Bromberg (1998) said that the goal for therapists is to maintain a bond with the client based on attunement to his or her subjective experience. Study respondents concurred. They stated that the affective traits of care, concern, and warmth communicated from their significant other were the most important factors in helping them to desist.

The main relationally based goal for clients to achieve from therapy is to gain the capacity for personal agency which incorporates the ability to make conscious decisions about behavior, to put those decisions into action, and to accept responsibility for those acts (Benjamin, 2010). Although the concept of personal agency obviously includes behavior, it also incorporates ego functions such as sense of self, decision-making ability, judgment, and the capacity for internalized conflict. Without it, actions become nothing more than compulsions (Stern, 2010), driven by unseen and incomprehensible forces which appear to be at once part of oneself and simultaneously alien.

For this practice theory, goals corresponding to the desistance process must also be included. Components of secondary desistance such as identity change, ownership of the desistance process, and a shift in the client's perception of his or her social status, must be incorporated into relational goals. Study respondents described their goal as "to become productive members of society." Relational goals which apply specifically to clients with presenting problems related to substance abuse, antisocial personality disorder (ASPD), and post traumatic stress Disorder (PTSD) are as follows:

1. For the therapist to establish and maintain a therapeutic relationship based on the affective qualities of care, concern, and warmth. The relationship must provide a safe environment to the client within which to share distressing self-states and behaviors. The goal of this relationship is for the client and therapist together to understand the subjective experiences of the client.
2. For the client to develop a decision-making process integrated among his or her major self-states, manage feeling states effectively without reliance on substances or criminal actions, communicate in words these inner states to him or herself and to others, perceive others as like him or herself, improve capacities for interpersonal relationships, and develop a cohesive sense of self capable of maintaining a prosocial lifestyle; together producing the ability to achieve and maintain secondary desistance and long-term sobriety.

Attachment

All psychotherapies and theories of social work practice, relationships specifically designed to facilitate change, begin with the common stance that the nature of the therapeutic relationship is one of the major agents of change (Fonagy, Roth, & Higgitt, 2005). The factors of therapeutic relationships common to all types of psychosocial intervention that create the capacity for change include empathy (Berenguer, 2007); hope (Snyder, 2002); positive regard (Farber & Lane, 2001); and motivation (Miller & Rollnick, 2002), all aspects of attachment.

In relationally based therapy, attachment is the cornerstone of therapeutic processes and operations. It serves to establish the relationship. It is a core building block of the therapeutic frame, a diagnostic mechanism, and an ongoing stance. Attachment is the instrument which enables the processes of internal exploration: witnessing, holding, and containment. It maintains the bond between client and therapist and mediates the distress brought on by these therapeutic functions.

The quality of therapeutic attachment also fuels both the entrance to and resolution of therapeutic conflict. Productive relationally based therapy brings forward dissociated self-states and unresolved trauma which leads to dissension. Attachment serves as a counterweight to the enormous pressure these conflicts place on the therapeutic dyad and as an anchor while the conflicts are rendered. As such, it is the crux of attaining and maintaining both sets of therapeutic goals.

Establishing a Therapeutic Relationship

An attachment-based therapy relationship has to be carefully established, nurtured, and maintained. The responsibility for this critical task falls squarely on the therapist (Bass, 2007) whose job it is to set and maintain the therapeutic frame, including its parameters or boundaries, emotional environment, and atmosphere of safe curiosity. Yet, engagement with this client population presents unique challenges.

The Client's Presentation All clients who apply for or are mandated to treatment do so due to defects, deficiencies, or inadequacies—personal failures of one sort of another. Thus, therapy begins with a power differential which is commonly a source of humiliation for clients. While it is difficult for anyone to realize a need for treatment and approach a new therapist, for substance abusing and offending clients, seeking treatment often further represents a history of failed interactions rife with negative judgment about their behaviors. Clients who are poor and marginalized by the larger community feel especially disempowered when seeking treatment. Mandated treatment further exacerbates these power differentials.

Furthermore, clients with pathology similar to that of the respondent group live in a state of crisis which conflicts with most service provision models, causing problems before client and therapist even meet. Entering treatment often constitutes a crisis for this client group because it indicates that they got caught engaging in an illegal activity. Additionally, they do not live scheduled lives. Remembering on which day and time an appointment falls and obtaining transportation to attend the meeting are tasks which may conflict with handling the crisis of the moment. Sometimes clients do not have private transportation. Often they do not have money to pay for public transportation or copays. Attending an intake appointment may be prioritized as secondary to obtaining money for drugs. Hence, late cancellations and no-shows are a frequent event.

In addition to the precipitant for treatment, clients bring their history of criminal offenses, substance abuse, trauma histories, character pathology, severe environmental stressors, as well as medical problems from the substance abusing lifestyle. Most likely, they also bring a history of failed treatment attempts. Clients with sociopathic traits assume others have the same motivation as they do: to get what they want in any way possible, to maintain control of interactions, and to reduce humiliation. When applying for treatment in a public agency, they expect to meet a therapist who is indifferent and overworked, someone who does the work solely for personal gain. These factors combine to produce conditions which can easily disable a first meeting.

Substance abusing and offending clients present themselves in a few set ways at the very beginning of treatment. They are either overtly hostile and suspicious, superficially charming and facile, demanding and in crisis, or a combination of these presentations. They arrive equipped with their arsenal of defensive maneuvers: hypervigilance about the therapist's motives, assessment of the therapist to determine the type and extent of manipulating they will try to accomplish, acceptance of nothing at face value, and a plan to predominate over the interaction. When clients try to control the therapeutic encounter, their goal is twofold. They are seeking to avoid being held accountable for their actions and to be relieved of any mandates such as ongoing treatment or urine screens. They also seek to gain concrete services or provisions such as psychiatric medication, medical appointments, or public transportation passes.

The Therapist's Self Therapists bring a self, personal experiences, and training that are very different from their clients in fundamental ways including psychological makeup; lifestyle, SES, values, and attitudes; and perhaps race, ethnicity, religion, and gender. Given the difficulties and differentials between substance abusing and offending clients and their therapists, it would seem easier for therapists to fall back on a generic, professional mode of interaction. The risk of doing so with this population is that the communication will fall flat. Clients who regularly do not tell the truth are especially sensitive to honesty in others' presentations. Anything less than an enthusiastic and caring approach will not come across as genuine. Ace described a treatment setting that seemed disingenuous to him and related how clients did not get what they needed from the agency.

> It was just a money-making organization. That's what I think of it. Just sending people right through, you know. They're not really catching on. They [treatment staff] don't care if they catch on or not. You had people that had been through there, been through the system three or four times. If they had teachers there to teach you, I mean, to really focus on your recovery, then you might get it. It's like a cycle. But they need the money. "So if we could just have you keep coming back, then we don't have to worry about our jobs."

Furthermore, in relationally based treatment, the attachment must be mutual. Clients must establish an attachment to their therapists in order for the work to unfold but therapists must also establish an attachment to their clients. Clients who do not feel genuinely cared about or important will not engage in honest and trusting self-disclosure. Therapists who do not feel an attachment to their client will not experience the bond necessary to hypothesize accurately about the client's problems, relational deficits, or dissociated self-states.

How does one approach this disheartening challenge? Basic psychodynamic training provides guidance on how to establish a therapeutic stance. Therapists learn to maintain evenly suspended attention between their own self and that of their client. They also learn to develop an observing ego to monitor interactions and exchanges. Modell (1991) described this ego function, unique to psychotherapists, as the ability to inhibit affective responses but not affective perceptions. These practices provide a boundary within which to situate oneself. Relationally, it is helpful to remember that the goal of treatment is to establish an affective attunement with the client. At this early phase of the treatment, it is helpful to look for something likable about the client and forge the initial attachment there until the therapeutic relationship is better established.

Certain characterological traits on the therapist's part are beneficial in this regard: an interest in engaging with clients from different walks of life, enjoyment of a challenge, a desire to help seriously ill people, comfort with verbally expressed anger, patience, and a sense of humor. Taylor, McMurran, and Riess (2007, p. 195) stated that "those who would help this group have to be highly skilled, very organized, and have a strong capacity for self-reflection on their work…" Mitchell (1993) offered an additional caveat. He stated that therapists treating aggressive clients have to embrace their own destructiveness before it can be transcended.

Limitations to Clients' Ability to Verbalize Adding to the challenges of the beginning of treatment, substance abusing and sociopathic clients are not able to articulate in words the full extent of their difficulties as the experiences and affects bound by dissociated self-states have been rendered mute (Stern, 2010). When first asked, study respondents could not articulate any of their internal states or reasons for their behavior. Although most attended 12 Step meetings and CBT-based counseling for substance abusers and offenders counseling, few had had the opportunity to engage in individual therapy and as a result, most did not have the words to describe their transitions.

When asked about their process of desisting from violent behavior, respondents stated that it was something they found they had to do although they often could not articulate their reasons, particularly when discussing the stopping and starting during their first attempts at sobriety and primary desistance. The following exchange with Ace is representative of how respondents first described their decisions and behaviors:

Q: How did you decide to go home then where you hadn't decided before?
A: I had too much. I just…I just had enough.

However, one of the questions on the interview schedule related to how much work respondents were willing to put into changing. Although respondents did not have the words to express their efforts, all 11 reported giving it their all. E said, "You work your ass off." Lee said that he works at it "constantly." Mark said that he did "whatever it took." Jay stated that his sponsor told him that "the only thing you have to change is everything." Respondents had learned the skills necessary to change their behavior but those in early desistance did not understand nor could they articulate what had changed internally to produce these new behaviors.

It was through the interview process that respondents were able to identify the factors affecting their transition. In response to questions and probes, they were better able to articulate the specific changes they experienced. Each respondent described how he was changed by his relationships so that he could perceive and experience himself and his life differently and thereby evolve from substance abusing criminal to sober community member. Some respondents were able to expand their capacity to verbalize and make sense of their journeys even within the very limited window of a one-time interview. Others were exposed to the benefits of this experience.

Why is being able to verbalize psychic and behavioral change necessary? At the most basic level, the process of therapy is talk-based. Poor and undereducated clients often do not have comparable verbal ability to those who had more advantages during childhood. Talking without a concrete purpose or to describe inner states may seem alien.

Furthermore, verbalization is the process that promotes self-cohesion. Without this ability, the capacity for personal agency cannot form because verbal processes integrate behavioral changes within the character. If clients are unable to describe to themselves or others why and how they are living their lives differently, their sense of self remains fragmented. Consequently, they would remain dependent upon what their significant others tell them to do. They would not know how to assess a situation, tolerate and manage affect, or make behavioral decisions.

Using the acquisition of language as a metaphor, those without adequate verbalization skills will only be able to repeat words or phrases told to them but not to formulate their own sentences based on their own ideas. Those respondents with over 10 years of secondary desistance and the most treatment were best able to articulate their intentions and reasons for their behavior. Therefore, one of the goals of relational therapy is to facilitate the client's acquisition of language with which to discuss his or her inner states.

Another obstacle to communication is that new clients also tend to be guarded and suspicious particularly if they are mandated to treatment by a state authority. Therapists represent the larger society and are viewed as agents of authority (Altman, 2005; Gaztambide, 2012; Harris, 2010). However, Skeem, Eno Louden, Polaschek, and Camp (2007) found that relationship quality in successful mandated treatment involved caring, fairness, trust, and an authoritative as opposed to an authoritarian stance. The affective aspects of the bond are critical to clients being able to take in the cognitive aspects of treatment.

The experience of genuine connectedness with an agent of authority also begins the repair process of the pain and humiliation of previous negative experiences. When clients are perceived as good by their therapist, the seeds of identification are planted. Hence at the beginning of treatment, the nature and quality of the therapist's attachment may be the only way for the client to assess the therapist's intentions and potential trustworthiness, to determine if the offer of therapeutic help is genuine, and to embark on this journey.

Tasks and Processes of Therapeutic Engagement

Assessment Given these obstacles to beginning a new treatment episode, assessment, which normally occurs at the first meeting, will be a difficult endeavor. Between clients' lack of ability to verbalize and their desire to minimize their previous behavior, much of what is said will not be accurate, leaving the therapist without much useful guidance with which to structure treatment. However, attachment can also function as a source of diagnostic clues. As the therapist reaches out to engage with this new client, he or she must allow the free flow of feelings to emerge in response to these attempts. An unattached and emotionally unengaged therapist will not be able to generate hypotheses about the sources of the client's affects and behaviors.

Starting the Therapy Process The affective nature of the therapeutic relationship provides the base for its core functions: witnessing, containment, holding, and identification. Lyons-Ruth (2005, p. 320) listed the necessary therapeutic actions which maintain this attachment:

1. A continuing attempt to learn the current subjective reality (affect state, current desired goal, and level of understanding) of the client
2. Giving responses that acknowledge that state
3. Ongoing construction and regulation of interactions
4. Remaining open to the entire array of affective communication
5. Both participants in balanced and mutually regulated dialogue
6. Negotiation and repairing of miscues, misunderstandings, and conflicts actively managed by the more advantaged partner (the therapist) to move communication toward more flexible and inclusive forms

Witnessing and Containment Attachment in relationally based therapy relationships is maintained by three therapist functions which occur simultaneously: witnessing, containment, and holding. In order for unformulated and severely traumatizing experience to be processed and made sense of, it is necessary to have another hear the testimonial and bear witness to the intense suffering experienced by the other. At once a concept and a process, Stern (2010, p. 111) described the impact of witnessing: "We need to feel that we exist in the other's mind, that this other is emotionally responsive to us, that he or she cares about what we experience and how we feel about it." Benjamin (2010) stated that understanding by another mitigates the suffering. It reinstates the sufferer's sense of the "lawful quality of experience" (p. 115) and with it comes the possibility of repair.

Unformulated experience in its unconscious form cannot be thought about. In sharing their stories, traumatized clients often present intense feelings of confusion about what happened to them. If these experiences occurred during childhood and were a product of a dysfunctional family, the client most likely suffered alone. Family members often deny what occurred or act as if it never happened, causing clients to be unable to make sense of their experiences.

Without another to process the experience, the trauma must be dissociated and relegated to a fragmented self-state (Stern, 2010) so that even within the character, the self-state holding the unformulated experience suffers alone. As a result, it is impossible to develop a coherent self-narrative. Bromberg (1998, p. 114) stated that "when life feels arbitrary, senselessly cruel, or meaningless one is liable to be aware of no story at all." The absence of a self-narrative prevents the ability to develop a coherent sense of identity.

The effects of unprocessed trauma on interpersonal capacities can be debilitating. Harris (2010, p. 725) described shame resulting from experiencing trauma as "a kind of giant systems crash, derailing and spoiling self and self in relation to others." A character structure riddled with dissociated self-states and no sense of ongoing identity is compromised in terms of its capacity for agency and intimacy. Close relationships would be approached with equal measures of need, wish, and fear.

The clinical task is to provide enough safety so that dissociated and unformulated experience can be expressed and conscious thought processes applied (Stern, 2010). The method employed to provide the witnessing function is containment, a concept introduced by Bion (1967). Containment is the therapeutic practice of managing intense affect between client and therapist. It is the therapist's task to tolerate the affect to the degree that it becomes bearable for the client.

Containment and witnessing as therapeutic processes serve to heal clients' emotional pain—permitting the reprocessing of dissociated and unformulated experience, improving cohesion of the sense of self, facilitating clients developing a more complete self-story or narrative, and improving interpersonal capacities. For clients with marginalized social status, therapeutic witnessing also provides a positive emotional connection to the larger society. Perhaps for the first time, clients encounter a member of this community who tries to understand and who accepts what they have been through. Their experiences are confirmed as painful and perhaps unfair.

Once the isolated trauma sufferer gains this witness who can contain the affect enough that it is rendered tolerable, the experience of the trauma becomes more possible to contemplate and understand. This capacity is called mentalization, a concept introduced by Fonagy (2001). Mentalization is defined as a reflective function which includes the ability to think through and accurately interpret the behavior of others and assign meaning to it. This capacity, a critical component of affect regulation, impulse control, self-monitoring, and personal agency, is a product of secure childhood attachments (Fonagy, 2001). When secure childhood attachments did not exist, the therapeutic process of witnessing can provide an adequate substitute. Client and therapist mentalizing together about the client's traumatic experience expands the client's capacities associated with personal agency.

When a therapist attends to a client's emotional pain, the witnessing process labels the client's experience as valid. Once the emotional pain can be brought forth in a safe and supportive interpersonal setting and formulated through mentalization, dissociation lessens. Telling the story of the trauma in this way integrates this aspect of experience into the conscious whole, strengthening the sense of self. Clients, seeing themselves differently and having been validated by their therapists, will be able to approach other interpersonal relationships from a less shameful and guarded stance. Benjamin (2010) explained that the repair process witnessing provides can reformulate the perception of relationship from dependence which was a "source of terrible pain and anxiety" (p. 115) to an experience of positive attachment.

This aspect of witnessing is especially salient for substance abusers and offenders who have rerouted their needs for emotional connection to the use of external mechanisms which mediate affect, including substance use and the illegal appropriation of money or material items. Dependence on people was most likely a source of humiliation and pain in which their needs went unmet. It is possible that engaging in a relationally based therapy may be the first time that clients experience their emotional needs being met within a non-traumatizing relationship.

When a therapist provides the witnessing function within a relationally based therapeutic relationship, the containment and processing of unformulated experience produce a joint outcome. The therapist will reframe, provide other ways of thinking about and feeling about, the traumatic experience based on his or her own training, experience, and character. Through the co-occurring mentalization process, the preexisting trauma and its sequelae, the experience of "not-me" in the presence of a caring and supportive other, and the therapist's responses about the situation become integrated and internalized within the client. The client's dissociated self-states formed about this trauma begin to dissipate as the understanding of the trauma is reconfigured. The now conscious material can be recalled and made sense of. Shame, rage, emotional pain, and distress are processed and consequently reduced.

An additional level of healing occurs for clients when those who are marginalized and disempowered share traumas with therapists who represent the larger society. Clients similar to study respondents will have experienced personal trauma that occurred within their families, cultures, and society, sometimes perpetrated by those representing the larger systems. Hence, clients bringing their personal stories of societal marginalization and disempowerment to the therapist's office would approach with wariness and suspicion. Altman (2005) stated that clients with a history of stigmatization and living in poverty view those representing the system as potentially both promising and rejecting. Therapists hold the promise of needed services but clients have also experienced negative judgment and rejection from staff of agencies providing these services.

When a therapist bears witness to the client's suffering at the hands of the larger society, the interaction provides a powerful counterbalance to the previous experiences. Several study respondents discussed how their pervasive distrust of members of the larger society changed as a result of therapeutic encounters. It sometimes took many years of treatment attempts before they realized as Bama said, "they just want you to do good." Any type of positive attachment with a representative of this culture and society will do much to heal these divisions.

Effects on the Therapist The powerful bond produced between client and therapist as a result of this healing process, a "mutual living-through" (Bach, 2006) has enduring effects on the therapist as well, some negative and some positive. Therapists can be touched by the nature of the client's traumatic experience and his or her distress in sharing it. The disclosures may trigger memories of the therapist's own traumas and combined with containing powerful affects for the client, the aftereffects may overwhelm the therapist's management capacity. Vicarious traumatization is a well-known and serious threat to the therapist's functioning (For an overview of the vicarious traumatization literature, see Williams, Helm, & Clemens, 2012). It is important for the therapist to be able to process any lingering effects with an experienced and capable supervisor.

Yet, therapists can also experience a sense of competence when witnessing succeeds at rendering dissociated states and reprocessing their clients' intense emotional pain. They may feel closer emotionally to the client after such an encounter. Furthermore, Iqbal (2015) suggested that vicarious traumatization could also lead to vicarious resiliency. Therapists may experience healing of their traumas from witnessing another's and a consequent strengthening of self and self-functions.

Holding Traumas and their sequelae must be relived in the present in order to be reprocessed but only to the extent possible within a safe and supportive setting. In order for witnessing to proceed, therapists must manage two tasks: to contain the negative affect and provide a holding environment during this process. Although these concepts are routinely treated as interchangeable within psychodynamic writing, they are separate functions. Holding applies to the therapeutic relationship on an ongoing basis. The therapist's goal is to maintain the integrity of the holding environment as much as possible throughout the course of treatment. Containment is a specific function employed as needed to detoxify negative affects or unformulated experience.

The concept of therapeutic holding, "ubiquitous in analytic work" (Slochower, 2005, p. 34), was first introduced by Winnicott (1958). He applied the concept of good enough mothering as it affects infant development to the task of the therapist who must provide an environment of safety, security, and trust for clients so that they can feel "held." This concept is the predecessor of what attachment theorists deem a secure attachment. It is also what study respondents described in their significant relationships: people who were not involved in drug abuse or criminal behavior; who were emotionally available, supportive, and reliable; who responded when study participants were in crisis; and who provided appropriate help.

The goal of the therapeutic functions of containing, holding, and witnessing is "to create an emotional space within which inner experience can be articulated..." (Slochower, 2005, p. 31). The three together are interdependent. Without maintaining the holding environment, witnessing will not be possible. Without witnessing, containment cannot be utilized to treat symptoms based on traumatic experiences because the trauma will not be brought forth. And without containment, the witnessing process will become overwhelming to both parties, perhaps retraumatizing the client.

Attachment provides the emotional underpinning without which any of these three clinical functions are possible. Together, they are the mechanism that can heal pain and render dissociated states. They provide a potent antidote to the overwhelming helplessness, solitary quality, and meaninglessness of traumatic experiences. They also provide the mechanism for identification.

Identification As witnessing, holding, and containment progress and the therapeutic engagement process strengthens, the client will begin to identify with certain therapist traits, methods of thought, or behaviors, and integrate them as part of his or her own character. Occurring at a subconscious level, the process of identifying with others results in important improvements in two psychological capacities. The first is the internalization of function, such as learning to self-soothe and gaining problem-solving and decision-making skills. The second involves the internalization of affective and cognitive capacities of the other that are integrated into the character (Gabbard & Westen, 2003).

Study respondents described that feeling accepted by a prosocial significant other with whom they had a strong attachment consciously created the desire to emulate that person. The two components of this process evident from their narratives were (1) identifying with significant others which led respondents to perceive themselves differently, conforming to the perceptions of their significant others; and (2) identifying with others in the community which led respondents to perceive others differently, causing a reduction in respondents' view of the larger community as hostile toward them. For clients with histories of serious substance abuse and criminal behavior, it is this twofold process detailed in Chap. 4 which begins the pivotal evolution to personal agency and identity change.

When therapists maintain a positive and hopeful stance toward clients and communicate through words, tone, and behavior that they are accepted and valued, clients can experience an improvement in self-esteem and a corresponding shift in their sense of self. The co-mentalization process that occurs during witnessing expands the client's perceptions, tolerances, and capacities. These processes combine to facilitate the client's internalizing some of the therapist's cognitive and affective capacities. The client's self expands and strengthens accordingly.

The second process of identifying functions interpersonally. Rather than seeing oneself differently, this shift involves viewing other people differently. The client begins to be able to perceive the therapist as a human being much like the client. This aspect of identification expands to include the larger society, as represented by the therapist, and enables the client to view others as people like himself. Respondents described two components of this process from their experience: (1) a new and positive perception of prosocial others from formal institutions such as the criminal justice system or treatment staff resulting from positive interactions with members of these organizations that realigns views of the larger society; and (2) the perception that others' pain is the same as their own: the capacity for empathy. The prosocial community comes to be seen as composed of people who are potentially kind and supportive and who experience pain as the respondent does. Interpersonal capacities are consequently expanded.

Clients who attend 12 Step meetings are encouraged to do volunteer work within the meetings as a way for them to identify with others who are sober. Clients, like study respondents did, may start to do volunteer work or work in the social services as a means of identification with their therapists. Volunteer work with "socially excluded groups" (Aresti, Eatough, & Brooks-Gordon, 2010) furthers a sense of belonging to the larger society, in turn improving self-esteem and creating additional identifications with prosocial others. As this process continues, negative perceptions of others, including representatives of the larger society and even those belonging to the CJ system, are diminished.

However, in contrast to the earlier discussion of the challenges of therapeutic engagement, the descriptions of witnessing, containment, holding, and identification give the impression that the therapeutic process is smooth sailing. Nothing could be further from the truth. The internal and external chaos inhabited by clients who are dealing with substance abuse problems and criminal behavior creates ongoing interpersonal chaos as well. Relationally, the therapist must enter the client's world in order to begin the therapeutic attachment process. Yet, even if entering this world is not the therapist's intent, from the very first moments of its inception, clients' experience of chaos will be imposed upon the therapeutic endeavor. In relational terms, therapeutic conflict takes the form of impasses, ruptures, and enactments.

Therapeutic Conflict: Impasses, Ruptures, and Enactments

In the normal process occurring during any therapy session, the give and take of discussion and exploration causes shifts in self-states for both client and therapist, with each self-state of each person responding to self-states of the other. These multiple self-states belonging to both client and therapist, ranging from healthy to pathological, create different pairings within the same relationship which each person experiences differently (Benjamin, 2009). Despite its seeming complexity, this ongoing system of interpersonal dialogue looks from the outside like a simple conversation. Dissociations happen on an ongoing basis between therapist and client, most of which pass without incident, perhaps even outside of the awareness of both parties. In these situations, holding is maintained.

Yet, the therapeutic holding environment is a fragile entity with many factors contributing to its instability. Intimacy produced by an externally imposed structure between relative strangers is difficult to experience, tolerate, or comprehend. The dynamic and mutually determined character of the therapeutic relationship creates constant change. The processing of dissociated and unformulated experience is by nature disruptive. Empathic attunement between two adults has its limits. Furthermore, the Winnicottian concept of the therapeutic holding relationship better represents the structure of the traditional psychoanalytic environment.

The differential structure of relational therapy compared to traditional psychoanalysis changes the character of therapeutic holding. From a relational stance, a mother with her infant baby in many ways does not approximate the interconnection between two unrelated adults, a therapist with training and experience and a client with "complex levels of awareness and conflict" (Slochower, 2005, p. 38) both of whom are active partners in the therapeutic endeavor. Although the nature of relational therapy may reduce the power imbalance between therapist and client, it cannot be entirely eliminated. The therapist is not all-powerful and able to provide for all of his or her client's needs as can a parent. The client may be disadvantaged but he or she is not a helpless infant. Viewing clients as the equivalent of infants is patronizing and contrary to relational tenets.

Furthermore, relational therapy with clients who have culturally defined behavioral problems places further pressure on the holding mechanism. Despite the therapist's best attempts, miscues, misunderstandings, and differences of opinion are frequent occurrences particularly when clients and therapists come from different worlds. Thus, the holding capacity, even if good enough, will inevitably fail (Slochower, 2005, p. 39). Relational therapists well understand the tenuousness of therapeutic holding particularly when applied to those with "multiple self-states and shifting states of identity powered by dissociative processes" (Harris, 2010, p. 711). When holding fails and conflict ensues, treatment termination is an unfortunate and common result. Either the therapist fires the client or the client fires the therapist.

Yet, disruption to the flow of the therapy is actually an inherent aspect of the process. If therapy goes smoothly, it is very likely that not much is changing, a type of enactment in its own right. However, not all disruptions are of the same quality or severity nor do they pose the same level of threat to the therapy endeavor. Although the terms "impasse," "rupture," and "enactment" are sometimes employed interchangeably, it is useful to distinguish them. For the purposes of this discussion, impasses are located at the mild end of the disruption continuum. Ruptures fall in the middle with enactments being the most severe type of conflict between client and therapist.

Impasses

Various types of impasses occur routinely due to the inherent power imbalance of the therapeutic relationship and cultural differences between clients and therapists. Misunderstandings, misattunements, and misreads by both parties are frequent events. They can consist of short stops; moments of incongruity that go unacknowledged. Or they may be misunderstandings of verbal content in which the conversation must be interrupted and the errors corrected. Overt disagreements may occur which must be addressed. Another example of an impasse is a cumulative sense by either or both parties that there is something wrong with the process of the therapy, something seems off, but it goes unarticulated. It is possible that all of these types of impasses might occur during a single session. Although many may remain unacknowledged, without resolution, impasses may become precursors to ruptures.

Ruptures

Ruptures are endowed with a dramatic quality and pose more of a threat to the therapeutic relationship than impasses. "A collapse of individual and dyadic functioning" (Harris, 2010, p. 721), ruptures are characterized by charged affective interactions usually involving anger, fear, or both. These crises "have a way of generating so much affect and consuming so much energy that one of the major problems becomes the disorientation of the therapist" (Russell, 2006a, p. 10). At this point, the stakes are raised to the point where the therapy itself is at risk (Bass, 2003).

Ruptures often involve breaches to the therapeutic frame, such as clients missing appointments frequently or no-showing, losing their temper during a session and behaving in an aggressive manner, or therapists refusing to help with a crisis-based request or demand. A client may withdraw by becoming silent, changing the subject, or being overly compliant or he or she may confront the therapist and become angry, blaming, or demanding (Safran & Kraus, 2014). Benjamin (2009) stated that ruptures feel as if the other is one's opposite pole; the doer versus done to. In this situation, neither can see the other's viewpoint nor does either feel heard. "It is as if the patient chooses the…potential rupture of the therapy relationship to try to convey that which is most important to him. And worse yet, he does so… by recreating the anguish for which he came to treatment to begin with" (Russell, 2006b, p. 10).

During ruptures, the client is overwhelmed. Although the therapist may be experiencing distress, it is tolerable and not causing a reciprocal dissociation. If therapists can avoid becoming rattled by this psychic assault, they are then free to think and feel their way through the attempted imposition of unformulated material and process these intolerable self-states with the client.

To do so, it is important to take a few moments to identify the feelings that the rupture engendered for the therapist which might include anger, disappointment, disorientation due to the abrupt nature of the shift, powerlessness to help this client, defeat, or inadequacy. These reactions could be understood diagnostically as non-verbal communications of the fragility and brittleness of the clients' self-states or as projections of the client's intolerable affects. The therapist is then free to formulate an intervention rather than react defensively. Ruptures, unlike impasses, cannot be ignored. They must be worked through; otherwise, they run the risk of precipitating premature termination.

Clinical Case Example

Mike was a 49-year-old married white male with four children ranging in age from 8 to 22. He was referred for outpatient counseling by the jail diversion program after he was arrested for assaulting his second oldest son, Keith, who was 15 at the time. Mike and his wife, Julia, had been struggling with Keith's behavior problems including criminal trespassing and vandalism; lack of attendance at school; and drug usage. During a confrontation, Keith lost his temper and pushed his mother to the floor. Mike punched Keith and threatened to kill him if he ever did anything like that to his mother again. Julia called the police. Keith was mandated to live outside the home until the court could determine if it was safe for him to return.

Mike had been in treatment several times in the past and had been diagnosed with PTSD. His parents had died tragically when he was young and he had been placed in foster care. He had never mourned these losses. Mike was alcoholic and used illegal pharmaceuticals when he could get them. He was indignant that the court was involved, insisting that he had every right to handle his family problems in any way he saw fit. He was incensed at his wife for calling the police, the police for arresting him, and the court both for removing his son and mandating Mike to treatment. It took many sessions of explaining the possible criminal justice implications before Mike realized that the court was doing him a favor. If Mike completed the counseling successfully as mandated by the jail diversion program, he would avoid incarceration and eliminate the arrest from his record. His initial response was that if anyone tried to lock him up, he would kill himself.

Because Mike had never before been mandated to treatment, he was suspicious about my role with the court. He was outright paranoid about the fact that the court supervisor had referred him directly to me, convinced that listening devices had been installed in my office by the court. I explained that I often received referrals from the court when there is a clear mental health component to the criminal behavior. I also explained the nature of the release he signed. I showed him the form I would submit to the court indicating only his attendance and general progress. It did not request information specific to anything disclosed in session. Beyond that, I did not try to assure him of the confidentiality of his treatment because I believed that doing so would only cause Mike to further question my veracity. However, I did make it clear to him that any aggressive behavior toward himself or others would not be tolerated.

Despite Mike's emotional instability, he was a good provider for his family. He loved his wife and children deeply but felt defensive and inadequate as a husband and father particularly after this confrontation with the criminal justice system. I met with Mike individually and in occasional couples meetings as I did not trust his report of what was going on at home. Julia was not afraid of Mike's angry outbursts and was committed to him. However, she was overwhelmed by his emotional neediness.

In the beginning of treatment, I felt it necessary to focus treatment on the issues which brought Mike to me: dealing with the court mandate, referring Mike for psychotropic medication, addressing his substance abuse, and helping him to keep control of his temper. Mike learned to trust me after a few instances in which I was able to predict how the diversion program coordinator would react toward him and helped him prepare the proper responses, thereby proving my allegiance to him. He did start psychotropic medication but it did not seem to have much effect.

However, my attempts to work on substance abuse and behavioral control backfired. The more I tried to focus on anger management techniques, the angrier and more agitated Mike became. At one point, after becoming quite angry and upset, he looked directly at me and said, "This isn't helping." So I stopped. Instead, I just listened to Mike complain about his frustrations. I felt somewhat stymied and inadequate as well as concerned about "letting go" of Mike's anger issues but after several sessions of this, he seemed to calm down and began to see the humor in situations. The more he laughed during meetings, the better he felt when he left and the better he managed at home.

So we found ways to laugh at the things and people that were angering him. When Mike would lose his temper at home, either he or his wife would call and I would talk him down. His drinking and drug use abated. Mike completed the jail diversion program several months later. His son was returned home. Keith graduated high school and started working as a laborer. Mike continued in therapy and as his anger stabilized, he became increasingly depressed. We explored his traumatic childhood and its long-term effects.

Later, as we began the termination process, we discussed the rupture as a turning point between us. Mike talked about the importance of being able to assert himself verbally and have someone listen and respond. He was able to articulate how in contrast, the events of his childhood had rendered him powerless. I explained that his lack of behavioral control was making me nervous. We both laughed about the fact that I had to calm down before he could. From this rupture, Mike learned how to ask for what he needed appropriately and started to take responsibility for his emotional states and actions. I learned that clients often know what is best for them and that for Mike laughter was his most potent anger management tool. I learned that my urgency about Mike's situation impeded my ability to focus attention on his needs.

Enactment

Thus far, much of this view of therapeutic conflict is consistent with traditional analytic concepts of repression, splitting, ego strength, and using countertransference as a source of diagnostic information. However, it is in the relational view of the countertransference process that the most variance from the traditional formulation occurs. Relationally, the therapist's responses are located as emanating from within him or herself rather than solely as a product of client pathology. They are viewed as a separate factor distinct from the client's provocation. This differentiation becomes paramount when exploring the concept of therapeutic enactments.

Enactments are a particular type of rupture. Relational theorists define them as consisting of two processes: dissociated self-states of the client erupting into consciousness and the therapist dissociating in response. They occur when the client's "not-me" states, previously cut off from human relatedness (Bromberg, 1998), are accessed within the course of a therapeutic encounter. Should a client's unformulated material touch upon a raw area of the therapist's and he or she dissociates as a result, there become two sets of selves who cannot hear each other (Benjamin, 2009). In this situation, the level of mutual disturbance is heightened (Holmes, 2011; Bass, 2003). Often, the enactment seems to be an attempt to deal by domination and submission with what is unconsciously felt to be unresolvable differences (Benjamin, 2009; Stern, 2010). Consequently, enactments produce the most risk to the therapy relationship.

However, from a relational perspective, enactments are not only unavoidable but also expected; they are "at once obstacles and opportunities" (Stern, 2010, p. 71) where "the interruptions are as important as what they interrupt" (p. 24). Since these most emotionally painful self-states are unformulated and cannot be expressed in words, the only means at a client's disposal is to communicate them through enactment (Benjamin, 2009; Davies & Frawley, 1994; Stern, 2010). The two most important aspects of enactments are their communicative function and the benefits to the therapeutic process of working them through.

D.L. Levit (personal communication, June 13, 2015) described two types of enactment: collision and collusion. Enactments of either a conflictual or collusive quality are both characterized by the absence of internal conflict (Stern, 2010). Neither the client nor the therapist experiences internal conflict about the interpersonal difficulties because each views the other as culpable. In conflictual enactments, the disagreement occurs between therapist and client. In collusive enactments, both parties act to avoid conflict entirely. Collision, the conflictual type of enactment, is louder and consequently more easily identifiable than collusion.

Collision During enactments of collision, there is an unconscious effort by the client to avoid experiencing self-states by trying to force the intolerable identity onto someone else, in this case, the therapist. The conflict that cannot be experienced within one mind is experienced as between or across two minds. Enactments of collision are a final defensive effort to interpersonalize dissociated material (Stern, 2010).

Stern (2010, pp. 119–120) stated that for those who have suffered severe trauma and whose vulnerability is therefore unmanageable, the eruption of "not-me" can be catastrophic. When "not-me" becomes "me," a precarious state of mind is suddenly created. He eloquently described the process as:

> 'Not-me' originates as a response to unbearable fear or humiliation, the experience of having been the object of a powerful other's sadism. It is the sense that one is once again that stricken person: terrorized and terrified, sometimes to the point of immobility or helpless, destructive rage; contemptible, sometimes to the point of a self-loathing that yearns for the destruction of self or other; shamed and horrified, sometimes losing the desire to live or creating the desire to kill; weak, sometimes to the point of a shameful and utterly helpless surrender that feels as if it can be prevented only by suicide or held at bay only by committing mayhem. One *will* not, *can*not be this person, because when one was, life was not bearable; and yet, if not-me enters consciousness, one *is* that person.

Mitchell (1993) discussed clients who are chronically aggressive as suffering from an enduring sense of threat and danger. He said that aggressive behavior in relationships is an attempt to protect the self from humiliation or insult and, as in Mike's case example, always feels subjectively justified. Furthermore, he stated that the physiological aspects of aggression make it difficult to contain. Its pervasive character serves to organize other self-states, making shifts to non-aggressive self-states more difficult. Aggressive stances by clients are also disturbing to therapists as they demand immediate containment.

Substance abusing clients maintain self-states whose function is to access external means with which to mediate affect. When they are sober and unable to access their coping tool, these clients are the least prepared to tolerate the affect generated by treatment conflicts. A client with a history of both aggression and substance abuse creates an ongoing challenge for the therapist to maintain holding and containment.

Davies and Frawley (1994) detailed three transference and countertransference positions that commonly occur during enactments with clients who have been sexually abused. It is my experience that these configurations also occur with clients with severe character pathology and PTSD.

1. The unseeing, uninvolved parent and the unseen, neglected child. When the client identifies with the parental position, the client is withholding and silent while the therapist is unwanted and unimportant. When the client identifies with the child, he or she is solicitous of the therapist and superficially compliant but ends up in an eventual rage.
2. The sadistic abuser and the helpless, impotently enraged victim
3. The idealized omnipotent rescuer and the entitled child

The first awareness therapists may have of their client's dissociated experience is through their own experience that the more they try to "understand," the more it feels as if they are off track and not maintaining affective attunement (Bromberg, 1998). When an enactment is operating, the verbal exchange feels stuck, lifeless, and pressured to the therapist. It suddenly feels very unsafe in the room, as if something just out of reach, unpleasant, and perhaps dangerous, were rapidly unfolding.

Eventually when these dissociated self-states erupt into consciousness, the effect is disorienting for client and therapist. Both may respond with emotional withdrawal and defensiveness (Benjamin, 2009). In what feels like a stunning turnaround, each has become an enemy working to scuttle treatment goals, suddenly unrecognizable, unknown, and perilous to the other. This mutual perception is accurate to some degree because the self-states of both client and therapist dominating these exchanges rarely have access to the conscious realm.

Stern (2010) described a relational form of projective identification where the client locates self-hatred as emanating from the other: "I am not contemptible-you are. You think I'm bad? No way, it's you who's bad" (p. 121). This exchange corresponds to Davies and Frawley's (1994) second transference/countertransference configuration, the sadistic abuser and the helpless, impotently enraged victim. The therapist then dissociates in response to this onslaught as his or her unmanageable self-states are called into consciousness.

What is most confusing for both client and therapist is that until it is rendered, delivered into consciousness, the meaning of the enactment remains inscrutable, happening over and over until conditions within the therapeutic relationship are such that it can be deciphered. With clients who have histories of substance abuse, criminal behavior, and severe trauma, the risks are great since responses to the enactment may involve self-destructive behavior, rage at the therapist, and/or matters of life and death. Here, the client is at his or her most vulnerable while the therapist is least able to respond therapeutically (Russell, 2006b). Affective attunement is impossible. Holding has been demolished. Witnessing and containment are detached and adrift.

Collusion As dreaded as these encounters may be, if this process does not occur, it is likely that the client is withholding significant aspects of him or herself in the service of avoiding problems or "protecting" the therapeutic relationship. Collusion works to avoid the emergence of conflictual material. Frankel (2002) explained enactments of collusion as indicators that both therapist and client view each other as an aggressor and consequently engage in "pacts in which each of us quietly agrees that neither of us will show his own real fear and vulnerability nor will we notice or expose the other's" (p. 134). This unconscious agreement corresponds to the first of Davies and Frawley's (1994) transference/countertransference configurations, the unseeing, uninvolved parent and the unseen, neglected child. Although the character of this therapy appears peaceful, therapeutic processes which facilitate change are as absent as they are during collisions. In this case though, rather than as the result of an overt conflict, it is the avoidance of the painful material that renders them unavailable.

Enactment Resolutions

Compulsive enactments of the affective fallout of traumatic events and relationships do not give the impression of being an aspect of therapeutic progress. In fact, it often feels more likely that they will never change and will succeed in destroying the relationship. The task of resolution appears insurmountable because the therapist is simultaneously being challenged and his or her own dissociated self-states are being activated. How do therapists move the conflict from interpersonal to intrapsychic space (Holmes, 2011) and facilitate the rendering of an enactment? Fortunately, an enactment provides all of the information necessary for its resolution.

Enactments are the most intense way in which the client relates with others and as such, it is imperative that they be shared within the therapy. Furthermore, enactments are one of most powerful methods of diagnostic assessment. They are considered to be windows to unconscious meanings held by the client (Lyons-Ruth, 2005) and a necessary means with which to access dissociated self-states (Bass, 2003) because the client is unable to communicate the dissociated material in any other way. The level of distress caused by enactments during the course of a treatment can be considered an accurate diagnostic indicator of the client's level of unformulated material, the amount and type of trauma suffered by the client, and the depth of his or her character pathology (Russell, 2006b).

During an enactment, the therapist will experience the affective imprint of what the client endured. It will permit the therapist to understand how and why the client's relational deficits came into being but more importantly, it will communicate the client's distress more effectively than any other method. Dissociated self-states are brought to the therapeutic relationship because they need to be healed and the client has hope that the therapist will be the one able to do this.

In order to do so, enactments must be recognized as they are occurring. This observation may seem self-evident given the distress level between therapist and client but since the therapist is dissociating and will likely find the distress level disorienting, he or she may be initially unable to comprehend what is happening. Once the process is labeled as an enactment, the therapist must recognize his or her own dissociative response and identify which self-states are being dissociated, and which thoughts and feelings are being cast from consciousness (Russell, 2006a). This is no easy task given the sudden and significant discomfort between client and therapist and the immediate demand to formulate a response, answer a request, and/or react to a crisis.

After identifying his or her self-states, the therapist then has to recenter. The self-state which predominated during the enactment must be acknowledged and set aside for later processing outside of the therapy. Attunement to the client's subjective state must be reestablished. The therapist can then focus attention on exploring the client's self-state(s) which produced the enactment and provide a witnessing function for this dissociated material. Once the enacted material is processed and contained, or rendered, it is transformed into an aspect of conscious character. This process may be accomplished in a matter of minutes, hours, weeks, or months, sometimes years, if it is a core aspect of self.

In order to utilize enactments diagnostically, the therapist must recapture his or her feelings as the enactment occurred. Some of those affective states occurred in response to the client's presentation while some of them represented painful aspects of the therapist's past (or present). It is necessary to differentiate them, to separate the client's issues from the therapist's. This is best accomplished with the help of a relationally trained supervisor or one's own therapist.

The therapist can then reconstruct the client's affective state as experienced by the therapist and gain a deeper knowledge of the extent of the client's painful experience; aspects that the client could not articulate. During the processing of the enactment, the therapist can share his or her experience of the dissociated material as a means to reconnect it with the client's previously unformulated material. However, this process brings up the thorny issue of therapist disclosure.

Therapist Self-Disclosure In most non-relationally based therapy, any personal disclosure on the part of the therapist is considered a breach of boundaries as the therapist's role is seen as one of participant observer. Normally, therapists use their training and experience to guide their client's progress but try not to disclose anything about themselves in the process. Since relationally based therapy is co-constructed and a mutual process, the therapist's role, boundaries, and type of engagement with the client are far more complex. It becomes imperative to share about oneself particularly in order to render enactments and yet, it is equally imperative not to derail the therapeutic process with material irrelevant or destructive to it.

In order to determine whether a disclosure is appropriate, its purpose must be clear. Disclosures are to be made only if the therapist is certain that they will expand the client's capacities or strengthen the therapy relationship. Using the differentiation process described above, the goal is to limit communication of aspects of the therapist's experience to that which occurred specifically with or about the client and to what is relevant to the therapy relationship.

Therapeutic Benefits of Rendering Enactments

When dissociated aspects of self are reprocessed and integrated, the conflicted material becomes part of the self. This constellation of thoughts, feelings, and memories are no longer foreign and can be experienced as emanating from one's own self rather than from the other. During the enactment resolution, the client can remember the conflict that occurred and hold the contradictory thoughts and feelings within him or herself. The relational exchange can be recalled and discussed calmly, with each party able to articulate his or her role in its formation. Both client and therapist learn more about the damage it represented. The dissociated material is thus freed from its solitary confinement while the therapeutic relationship is released from its polarized standoff. Client and therapist can both see themselves and each other more clearly. Powerful change has occurred.

Benefits to the Client The benefits of this process to the client are substantial including both interpersonal and intrapsychic gains. Interpersonally, the client would experience the reduction of painful affects, feel validated and supported in his or her efforts, and feel understood and accepted in a profound way by the therapist, a very different experience from the collision of his or her conflicting self-states.

As the client's self expands to incorporate dissociated material, a salient, although painful, aspect of experience becomes part of the client's character. Important parts of the self are no longer exiled. Dissociated aspects are returned to their rightful places, allowing the client to take ownership and responsibility of them, experience warded-off pain, and mourn losses (Holmes, 2011). Hence, from a relational stance, cognitive understanding follows this intrapsychic change. It does not create it (Boston Change Process Study Group, 2013).

The client's sense of internal emptiness is reduced. Mental energy expended to maintain dissociative areas as separate is freed to be used for conscious activities. Feelings of competence are increased as helplessness and despair are reduced because the traumatic experience has been drained of its destructive power. The ability to see and articulate aspects of life, self, and problems grow and therefore, the client's self-capacity is expanded (Stern, 2010).

Benefits to the Therapeutic Relationship The rendering of an enactment shifts therapeutic processing to a more complex level because the client experienced further integration of dissociated selves. Each time an enactment is survived with the therapeutic relationship intact, the client experiences a contrasting experience from the course of the traumatic event that caused the original dissociation. The client was able to expose and bear his or her feelings with another person in a safe environment, thereby reducing suffering and enhancing self and mutual regulation (Benjamin, 2010). As each pathologically dissociated self-state comes into awareness through a relationship with another person, interpersonal safety is reinforced and emotional intimacy is strengthened. The painful affects of the self-state, too great to tolerate alone, were held between the client and therapist momentarily. "The safety of aloneness is gradually, very slowly, relinquished in favor of an utterly new event: safety within a relationship" (Russell, 2006a, p. 44).

Relationally, clients learn that conflict does not have to permanently damage or destroy a trusted bond. They do not have to offer themselves to be victimized nor do they have to take the role of aggressor. They find other relational capacities not limited to victim–victimizer typologies. They learn to express in words. They learn to do what the therapist did: hang tough, remember the attachment, and access their other self-states. They learn to have faith that the relationship can be repaired and that the client is important and valuable enough for both of them to fight for the relationship. Seriously divisive issues can be worked out and close relationships can be a source of healing and growth. The past internal schemas and relational patterns are flexed and changed. Their story is rewritten. The enactment process and language can be referred to and used as a marker for further therapeutic growth and work.

Benefits to the Therapist For the therapist, rendering an enactment is a validating and empowering experience. The client was retained in treatment and the therapy process rescued from a possible disruptive, damaging, and inappropriate termination. The therapist gains important information about the client's past experiences and the depth of his or her pain. The growth and consolidation that takes place in the wake of a successful resolution of an enactment can be stunning.

The therapist's self is also strengthened as a result. The enactment forced to consciousness an area of difficulty that had been dissociated for the therapist. In order to recenter, that area had to be identified and processed. The therapist's self expands accordingly as does his or her competence at locating and differentiating aspects of self that should either be withheld or shared with the client. This feeling of competence reduces anxiety during future enactments, serving to remind the therapist during these distressing interactions that they can be utilized for therapeutic benefit.

Clinical Case Example

Edward was a 36-year-old married African American male who was incarcerated for manslaughter. At a time and place in the distant past when inmates were able to access mental health treatment, Edward and I met for weekly individual therapy. Beginning with our second meeting, Edward would begin the session with a request to call his wife (Pay phones were available in the cellblocks for personal calls and departmental policy precluded inmates' use of phones in the Mental Health Department unless it was an emergency).

Each week I explained the department policy and would remind Edward that making phone calls was not the purpose of our meetings. I attempted to explore why he wanted the call and why he would ask each week when I always refused, all to no avail. Edward's only response was that he believed I was trying to provoke him into a rage. Although the exchange would only last several minutes, he would refuse to engage verbally, become extremely angry, and stare at me coldly for what seemed like hours. Eventually, Edward would begin talking about other issues and would stay for the duration of the appointment. And he returned each week.

Despite feeling perplexed and placed off balance by the demand, I was able to form an attachment to Edward. He was honest about his crime and his psychiatric and drug abuse history. He tried very hard to impress me that he was better than what he perceived was a typical inmate. For example, he tried to use complicated vocabulary when talking to me but unfortunately, he did not use the words correctly. I could strongly sense his humiliation at being an incarcerated client.

For me, the enactment brought up feelings of confusion and helplessness. What did it mean? What was it holding? I did not feel personally threatened nor did I fear Edward would lose his temper but I dreaded this weekly exchange. I had no idea what he wanted. Was this a sociopathic ploy to see if I would break the rules and give him what he wanted? And what would it mean to him if I did? Why was it always a call to his wife? Did he want me to be impressed with his attempts to remain in contact with her? Did he need the reassurance of her voice when facing the meeting with me? Was he worried she would leave him? Did he just want another opportunity to talk to her? Given his refusal to answer the first set of questions, I chose not to ask these. I did not know what else to do each week except to repeat the enactment. It became the ritual with which we began each session. At one point after several months, I gave up trying to understand it.

And then one day at the beginning of this particular session, Edward made his request to call his wife. I sadly shook my head no. Then he said, "I guess the reason I am down here is to talk about myself and not to make phone calls, huh?" A small smile appeared in response to my look of stunned relief. He never asked again and with that, the enactment was rendered. However, I was left being unable to understand the meaning of this struggle.

At the most conscious level, the request appeared to be an attempt to discover if I really wanted to talk to Edward, to see if he was acceptable to me. At a deeper level, it could be that the therapy prospect scared Edward and in response, at the beginning of each session, he created conditions which caused me to feel a parallel sense of uncertainty. It also could represent the dynamics of Edward's relationships. I knew that despite his best attempts, Edward's ability to express himself verbally was limited. I imagined a little boy desperately needing things from his parents who would respond by becoming enraged and then blaming Edward for their response. I also imagined people making demands of Edward that he could not meet, his becoming enraged, and being blamed for it. I imagined Edward not understanding the purpose of an interaction, asking for something he wanted, and both parties becoming angry. As our ritual continued to occur, I continued to contemplate.

Over time, I wondered if the enactment represented his offense. Edward had described the manslaughter as occurring in a nightclub. He said that the man he killed was the friend of a friend who had made obscene gestures and provoked Edward for no apparent reason. Edward calmly reached for his weapon and killed him. His history of PTSD and his explanation of events led the prosecution to charge him with manslaughter, a non-premeditated killing.

I tried to reconstruct the event based on my affective responses. Edward had responded to my denial of his demand to call his wife with the statement that I was trying to provoke him into a rage. I found the exchange bewildering but I knew that he had been provoked into a rage preceding his offense. I dreaded and feared our beginning interaction. I was not trying to provoke him. I was only setting my boundaries where they were supposed to be. I was shocked and scared by his response but I did not feel overtly threatened.

I began to have a sense that this was Edward's affective experience when he was confronted by his eventual victim. Edward was at the bar with his friends. He engaged with someone he thought was a friend who became enraged and reacted in a bizarre manner that Edward was not expecting. He felt attacked and scared and felt he needed to set a boundary with this person. However, he had also been triggered by the response and so could not determine the level of danger. He reacted based on past traumatic events and killed the man. Through the enactment, I was able to imagine some of Edward's affective states and hypothesize what he had experienced during his offense in a way that he could not communicate in words.

I categorized this as an enactment and not a rupture because the exchange was so stuck and it went on for so many months. Additionally, there were aspects of my responses that felt dissociated to me. In one way, my questions were attempts to reduce my own anxiety about the encounter between him and me, to preemptively resolve it so I could avoid the difficult affects. Because the questions were based on my own needs, perhaps my attempts to "understand" our enactment felt like assaults to Edward. Perhaps he feared that I would try to kill him, that he would be destroyed by the therapy attempt. He said he felt deliberately provoked by me. Perhaps he was afraid he would lose his temper again. Perhaps I was afraid of my anger at him. When I let go of trying to impose my questions on the process, he shifted his stance.

Several months after the phone call requests had stopped, I asked Edward what they had been about. He shrugged off my question. I was sad that Edward chose to avoid talking about this with me and believed it indicated that some of the beneficial aspects of the enactment's rendering were unrealizable. This felt like a parallel to the original enactment. However, I could also see evidence of Edward's significantly improved functioning. I felt that Edward was choosing to maintain a distance from me by not engaging in that process. Given our cultural differences, his incarcerated status, and limitations to his ability to verbalize, I accepted being unable to understand his reasoning and I resolved to respect his decision.

Capacity for Internal Conflict

The rendering of enactments produces the achievement of internal conflict for the client (Stern, 2010), one of the most important self-functions to be gained (Bromberg, 1998). When competing self-states are unaware of each other, an internal sense of conflict does not exist and the person will simply lurch from one self-state to the next while being unable to articulate reasons for his or her contradictory behavior. Enactments force conflicting self-states to consciousness and the rendering process permits these states to become articulated, mentalized, and integrated.

The treatment attempts of primary desistance are an example of a lack of capacity for internal conflict in which dissociated, opposing, and contradictory self-states vie for control. Active addictions are the result of opposing self-states in which the "me" and "not-me" of using versus abstaining switch in and out of consciousness. The client's addicted self-states sometimes yield to those that desire to abstain and be sober. However, those sober self-states are brittle and weak. When the client is overwhelmed by negative affect or stress, the sober self-states cannot cope. They recede to the subconscious as the addicted self-states come forward to mediate the affect and prevent the client from becoming overwhelmed. Much unformulated and painful mental material, most likely created by traumatic experiences and relationships, produce these rigid, split self-states characteristic of personality disorders. This personality organization does not have the strength to maintain sober behavior.

The ability to experience internal conflict is critical to the therapy endeavor because without it, therapeutic guidance cannot be taken in and integrated within one's character. Self-states representing the full range of behavior must be consciously accessible in order for clients to hear and accept ideas concerning behavioral change. From a relational perspective, it becomes very clear when addicted clients are without a capacity for internal conflict.

In this case, the abstaining self-states are most likely present during therapy sessions and passionately expressing thoughts and feelings about the need to abstain. The addicted self-states, while unable to articulate their needs in words, maintain control of behavior. Without internal conflict, a client can sit in a therapy session and express his or her desire for abstinence in a genuinely heartfelt manner. However, once out the door, the other self-states take over and substance abusing behavior resumes.

Clients without the capacity for internal conflict are not able to express in words why or how these shifts occur. When treating clients who also engage in criminal behavior, it is easy to mistake the disjunction between spoken words and actual behavior as indicative of sociopathy, concluding that the client is simply telling the therapist what he or she wants to hear while not experiencing remorse about the dysfunctional behavior. Yet, it is impossible to gauge the client's level of remorse until these self-states integrate.

Guidance and Confrontation

Clients attempting sobriety and avoidance of criminal behavior need a tremendous amount of guidance from prosocial others to learn to manage even the most routine stressors and problems without resorting to previous coping strategies. Without the capacity for internal conflict, guidance and confrontation from therapists about dysfunctional beliefs and destructive behavior will be experienced as narcissistic assaults, causing humiliation, anger, and suspicion. If only the sober and prosocial self-states are consciously accessible and present, the client can become morally outraged that the therapist does not believe that he or she will be able to manage the task. If only the addicted self-states are present, the client summarily rejects the guidance because these self-states do not want to desist.

In either case, typical responses include client withdrawal, pseudo-compliance, ruptures, passive aggression, or early termination, making it impossible to teach clients what they need to know to change their states of mind and behaviors. However, once this capacity is achieved and clients can locate the conflict about problem behaviors as emanating from within themselves, they can hear their therapists' thoughts about their behavior and thinking processes without becoming defensive.

At the time of the interviews, study respondents were unanimous in declaring their need for guidance from others. However, their level of dependence on outside advice and feedback varied based on the amount of time in which they had practiced these new skills and capabilities. It seemed evident that those in early desistance had less ability to experience internal conflict than those with many years of sobriety and crime-free behavior.

Mark, who decided early on in his criminal career to desist, described his experience of learning to assess his own his dysfunctional thought process from guidance and confrontation received in treatment. It is clear from his description that he was able to simultaneously be aware of the contradictory self-states of wanting to engage in criminal behavior while experiencing the need to let it go.

> I learned once I got to the program that the way I thought [chuckling] was absolutely insane. They did what was called Thinking Reports. You write down a situation and then you write the thoughts that you had with it, the feelings that came with it, and the outcome. And I would do a Thinking Report and I'd be thinking, "Damn! Who did I think I was?" [Both laughing.] I had this thinking like I could do whatever I want whenever I wanted and that's just the way it was.

Those respondents in early desistance reported that they needed continual access to the source of guidance because they did not yet have the capacity to internalize it as their own cognitive skill set. However, it was only from those with whom they had a strong attachment that they could hear the guidance they so needed. And even with that level of attachment in place, respondents with little capacity for internal conflict continued to experience the confrontation as a challenge to their self-esteem.

Black was the only member of the respondent group who moved to secondary desistance without the benefit of treatment. Although he had been drug and crime-free for 4 years, he described significant dependence on his wife to monitor his behavior and give continual encouragement, guidance, and confrontation about poor thinking, impulsive behavior, and the reasons to remain sober and crime-free. He struggled to accept her guidance while being unable to generate this process from within himself.

She came home one day and I had a bunch of weed that one of my friends had and I was like, "I'm just going to sell this." And she was like, "And then what? You know what I mean?" And I'm like, "That's just so we can have some money and we can start" because she was working and "we can get out of here quicker, I could just sell this a few times." And she was like, "You know that's not going to work" and I'm like, "Well you know, at least we can have what we need." And she was like, "It's not gonna work. It's not even worth the risk of you trying to do that and then what? The little money we got saved, you go out there and try to sell this, and you get arrested and then we back to square one because now I've got to give up our money that we've got saved to try to get you out of jail." That's my reality, she's my reality check because she keeps me focused. She keeps me grounded.

Q: And you let her keep you grounded.

A: Yes because I'm not used to letting anybody be in control. I'm always, it's always about me. I always got to be in the driver's seat. And my best thinking always gets me locked up [laughs] so you know I've got to let somebody else do.

Once the capacity for internal conflict is established, cognitive-behavioral methods of intervention can be taught to the client. However, these methods and confrontation about dysfunctional states of mind and behavior must emanate from within a caring relationship. Confrontation without care results in anger and defiance. This stance corresponds to Davies and Frawley's (1994) second transference/countertransference position of the sadistic abuser and the helpless, impotently enraged victim. Alternately, however, care without confrontation results either in enabling or collusion in which self-states attached to substances and criminal behavior are ignored. This stance corresponds to the third transference/countertransference position of the idealized omnipotent rescuer and the entitled child.

Collusion and Enabling In this culture, dependence on others is considered a personal defect, which when experienced, results in a sense of inadequacy. More "helping" results in more inadequacy. Those who are being "helped" and who have insufficient coping strategies to manage negative affect will rely on further acting out behavior to reduce these increasing feelings of inadequacy.

Rage often results when others perform tasks or functions of which the person is capable. Why? Because those being enabled know the enabler believes them to be incapable. Additionally, enablers impose their view of what they want from the other. Their goal is to fashion the enabled person into whom they want him or her to be, regardless of the enabled person's preferences, all in the guise of providing care. When the enabled person is unable to articulate what appears wrong about this care, the frustration causes a reversion to expressions of rage.

When people are enabled by others to engage in self-destructive behaviors such as drug abuse, additional meanings are construed. The enabler is avoiding conflict and succumbing to what the enabled person says he or she wants although the enabler is well aware that it is wrong to do so. Those who enable give in to the demands not because they think their intervention is going to help but because they tire of dealing with the conflict. It is a way to get the enabled person to stop making the demands, a passive aggressive maneuver.

Another reason for enablers to encourage destructive behavior is that doing so permits those with a shaky sense of self to organize themselves around the needs of the enabled. An example is a parent who continues to support an addicted and criminally involved adult child living in his or her house. These parents often present as being obsessed with what the child is doing and desperate to get it to stop and yet they give in to the child's demands ostensibly due to fear that if they refuse, the child will get in more trouble or die. They tend to minimize or deny their children's behavior and seem shocked when it recurs. Enabling parents give the impression of sacrificing their own lives to take care of their child, while in fact they are enabling the child to continue the dangerous behavior. In this manner, parents avoid managing troubling feelings and other issues in their own lives.

In any of these situations, because the primary purpose of enabling is to avoid conflict, enabled people know their enabler is unwilling to fight for them. Hence, enabling of another actually entails a rejection of that person. Firstly, it is an attempt to fashion the person into someone he or she is not. When the attempt is unsuccessful, the enabler accedes to the demands as a way to dismiss the enabled person. Enablers believe they are showing or providing care by this behavior but in actuality, enabling manifests a lack of relational capacity.

Therapists enable their clients in two main ways which both serve to avoid the client's negative affects and behavior. Firstly, therapists complete tasks for clients that they need to learn to do for themselves, either to avoid clients' demands or to calm their distress. Secondly, therapists make the mistake of maintaining a sole focus on the client's sober self-states and collude with the client, acting as if his or her addicted self-states have disappeared.

Therapists who seek to fix clients' problems focus on the stressors in their lives instead of the clients' responses to these stressors. They mistakenly believe that relieving clients of these problems will eliminate addictive coping strategies. What has actually occurred is the transfer of responsibility for the client's life and life choices to the therapist, who is unable to control what the client does. In this scenario, the client will become increasingly dependent on the therapist to take care of problems. This is not guidance. Doing for others does not teach them the skills to manage on their own and consequently, dysfunctional behavior will not be reduced by this stance. In fact, it may increase.

The second common way to collude with clients is to avoid addressing their negative behavior. Here, sole focus is maintained on self-states active in the treatment process while those aspects of the client's character that remain attached to substance abuse and criminal behavior are ignored. The capacity for internal conflict, if present, is not utilized because only one set of self-states are the focus of treatment. Much cognitive and behavioral information can be transmitted in this case but it will not be integrated within the client's character.

As the process of therapy becomes subverted to meeting therapist and client needs to avoid these conflictual areas, the identification process is similarly subverted. Clients will identify with the therapist's need to ignore their negative self-states while their own desire to avoid dissociated self-states will be reinforced. Hence, treatment goals are sacrificed. This form of collusion produces a client who appears far more functional than he or she actually is.

Clients with a lot of treatment experience, who know what to say and when, who present themselves as articulate and "getting" the program, can easily act as if they are the program "stars" without the commensurate ability to control their behavior. E described a period of time in which treatment staff believed him to be sober and capable and gave him inappropriate responsibilities as a result.

> So it was 6 months inpatient and 18 months outpatient. I got through that, not sober but I got through that. Once I got out of the inpatient, I came back to this area and was living in a sober house. I started drinking probably two months after I got there. I became the president of the house and the president of the chapter of **** Houses. And drinking the entire time I was there. That lasted for about 18 months. And then I was starting to shoot heroin and cocaine again. I couldn't mask that behavior very long. They caught on to it. I got asked to leave.

E was permitted to progress quickly because treatment staff was not able to glean the existence of his other self-states unaffected by his treatment attempts. It may have been that this negligence was partially a product of staffing and budget pressures as well.

While providing guidance, it is incumbent upon the therapist to assess the client's capacity for internal conflict and ensure that all of the client's self-states are represented during the therapy. If the client does not have a capacity for internal conflict and if all therapeutic time is spent on developing cognitive coping skills, the addicted and criminally involved self-states can gather strength because they are being ignored in the treatment. As Rothschild (2010, p. 141) described:

> For example, the phrase "that's my disease talking" frequently represents a way of dismissing what may be valid feelings arising from the desire to use. In this kind of treatment, rather than silence the wish, we actively engage with it and find out what purpose(s) it serves and how we can meet its needs without dangerous substance use. If the client believes that the therapist does not want to hear about a desire to use, or that it is dangerous or wrong to speak from that place, the client may agreeably go along with learning tools for sobriety without articulating doubts about wanting to use them.

Equal measures of caring, guidance, and confrontation at this point in the treatment process carry the best means with which to effectively address dysfunctional behaviors. A strong therapeutic attachment will function to continue the witnessing and containment of dissociated self-states. It will also provide the therapeutic "glue" to weather ruptures and enactments. The client will experience identifications with the therapist and internalize his or her strengths and skills. CBT-based coping tools can be provided as additional forms of guidance. Combined with the capacity for internal conflict, these new capabilities and skills produce personal agency.

Personal Agency

From the internal experience of conflict, the self expands to be capable of personal agency. This capacity comprises self-management: the ability to make conscious decisions about behavior, to put those decisions into action, and to accept responsibility for those acts (Benjamin, 2010). Stern (2010) described personal agency as, "the mind can feel and reflect on what it could only live out blindly before" (p. 103).

However, internal conflict may not feel like an achievement to clients experiencing it for the first time. The illusion of a cohesive sense of self is maintained when conflict is externalized. Denial about substance abuse also maintains self-deception about behavioral control, exemplified by the commonly heard statement, "I can stop whenever I want." The compulsive nature of crime and addiction reinforces itself. These rigidly structured processes feel more clearly defined than the murky cacophony of multiple internal voices representing the conscious and contradictory self-states created by internal conflict.

Yet, as internal conflict evolves into the capacity for personal agency, clients begin to experience a newfound sense of self-determination including control over behavior, belief in their freedom, and the ability to assume responsibility for their own actions and inactions (Benjamin, 2010). Others' guidance, so needed during earlier phases of therapeutic work, begins to be internalized and integrated within the client's own character. In contrast to action based on impulses and addiction, the behavioral control that emanates from personal conflict feels as though it belongs to oneself. It emanates from the inside rather than being either sought or imposed from outside. The capacity for personal agency permits multiple options for problem resolution based on open thought processes rather than the closed system of addiction and its default response of compulsive behavior.

Mental energy needed to enforce dissociation of self-states is freed to be used for other previously impossible but important mental processes including self-assessment and self-reflection. Personal agency permits the capacity for introspection–the ability to observe one's own mental and emotional states and insight–the ability to understand these states and what affects them (Gabbard & Westen, 2003). Furthermore, being able to reflect about one's own state of mind allows one to cognitively process in the present, as events are transpiring (Bromberg, 1998).

Self-assessment strengthens judgment, decision-making, impulse control, and other integrative functions of the self. These strengths and capacities allow for initiative (Stern, 2010), the ability to set a goal, determine the direction and actions to take, and achieve it. Clients move from simple avoidance of substances and criminal behavior based on external demands or repercussions to an internally motivated set of behaviors. Pink Panther described it as:

> The only way I will go back and relapse is if I want to. It's not like someone telling you. It's my decision because no one can make me do any anything that I don't want to do within myself; it's up to me. That's the way I look at it. I used to take the easy way out. Somebody says something wrong to me, or she done or say something wrong, I'd go get me a bottle to medicate myself. And then after it's over with, everything is gone. It's just the problem is still there, you know what I mean? I'm a much stronger person than how I was three to five years ago.

The capacity for personal agency may occur in phases. Over half of the respondent group curtailed violent behavior first before they tackled polysubstance addiction and its associated criminal behaviors. Given the enormity of the change necessary to achieve full abstinence from substances and criminal behavior, clients may renounce groups of behaviors sequentially rather than simultaneously.

Although cause for celebration, these new capacities and mental organization can cause anxiety. The therapeutic focus during the emergence of personal agency should be directed at managing both the cognitive and affective spheres. Clients need help to learn these new cognitive processes; to be able to identify and label them, understand their use, and practice them in session. Therapists can certainly provide

CBT-based material as well as their own judgment and decision-making capacities for modeling purposes but it is crucial not to impose their own thought processes or solutions as doing so may entail enabling. Clients would then regress to depending upon others for guidance or resort to impulsive behavior. Clients' anxiety levels should be closely monitored as they venture into this new territory. Affect management and coping strategies should be combined with cognitive skills to help the client avoid becoming overwhelmed as well as ensuring the integration of these new skills.

Newly found personal agency also places great stress on interpersonal relationships. This capacity reduces conflicts with others because as the guidance function is internalized, the need for confrontation is lessened. It would seem that this change should improve relationships. However, as disorienting as the capacity for personal agency can be for the client, it can also cause anxiety and confusion for his or her significant others. Those who have supported and cared for the client during the years of dysfunctional behavior are not accustomed to this new person who can take responsibility for his or her behavior. Trust sometimes takes a long time to achieve and clients can become confused and angry when their significant others do not happily embrace their new prosocial sense of self. Additionally, dysfunctional relationships based on enabling or controlling the client will begin to implode.

Macrolevel relationships change as well. Achieving the capacity for personal agency begins the transition from primary to secondary desistance. The experience of personal agency may feel alienating to those whose identities were based on membership in substance abusing and criminal subcultures. Clients come to realize that in order to fully change their behavior, they must forego their connections with their former compatriots.

12 Step programs provide a critical function by furnishing a transitional social membership. Association with sober 12 Step members allows for a new network of sober friends and sponsors and yet who also represent one's former life. Clients can speak at meetings about their former activities and lifestyle in a context of understanding and acceptance but that does not condone it. Relational capacities gained through the therapy process aid clients to meet new kinds of people who are sober and law abiding and to engage in new kinds of relationships with these new people.

Identity Change

For many clients who do not belong to subcultures based on destructive behavior, the achievement of personal agency marks the culmination of therapeutic work and the transition to the termination phase of treatment. But clients who have lived their lives as substance abusers and offenders must forego membership in their previous communities and join the larger society. Almost all study respondents indicated that they had to change their sense of their identity from that of criminal to sober and prosocial community member in order to completely abstain from illegal behavior. They had to be able to see themselves as productive members of society in order to limit their behavior to prosocial activity.

In what may seem like a chicken-and-egg argument over which came first, it possible that abstention from negative behavior caused identity to shift and not the other way around. However, based on respondents' narratives, attachment to significant others who could perceive the good in them brought about their ability to identify these traits within themselves. For them, the attachment-based change in self-perception preceded the ability to change behavior.

Moral Development

Identity transformation requires learning and internalizing a new set of values pertaining to how to treat others. Because substance abusers and offenders so often impose their addictions on their significant others through theft, domestic violence, and emotional abuse, they must learn to value and respect others as they learn to value and respect themselves. This system of morality must assign the values of right and wrong to thoughts, behaviors, and events and must be enforced by a functional and internalized sense of guilt. Over time, the morality system should include genuine remorse for past offenses. Brother Nowapo's tale of the murderer, "One Handprint Closer to a Change of Heart" recounted in Chap. 2, illustrated the necessity of moral guidance in order to renounce violent behavior and become a better person so that after death, one's soul might ascend to heaven.

As discussed in Chap. 5, it is often said that sociopaths have no conscience. It is my experience that substance abusers and career criminals only behave as if they have no conscience. They do have an internalized sense of right and wrong but it does not affect their behavior because their conscience is located within their sober self-states. Guilt emanating from a sober self-state will be as rigidly construed and brittle as the sober state itself. Any guilt a client with sociopathic traits consciously experiences becomes overwhelming and must be reduced or eliminated by continued substance abuse or criminal behavior. Once the capacity for internal conflict is achieved and the client is engaged in an identity change process, remorse and guilt become tangible. Therapists need to assess on an ongoing basis the client's capacity to tolerate these feelings.

Alternately, psychopathic clients do not have an internalized sense of right and wrong. A client's psychopathy will become evident during the middle phase of relationally based therapy, particularly during witnessing. He or she would describe what would sound like traumatic situations but the dissociated affect would not appear or if it were produced, it would not come across as genuine. This client would be unable to connect interpersonally or engage affectively in the therapy process. After the initial period of charming presentation, as the demands of therapy increased, the psychopath may become increasingly angry and demanding. No amount of processing would be successful at resolving it. Once the determination was made that his or her goals were unattainable, the psychopath would stop attending.

Clinical Case Example

David was a 34-year-old African American male with a long history of incarcerations, drug abuse, and violent and non-violent behavior, who was serving a 10-year sentence for robbery. His outside relationships seemed based primarily on intimidation. Inmates were afraid of him due to his violent and erratic behavior. He requested therapy to work on his anger.

After some initial testing of me, his behavior settled down. David stopped getting disciplinary reports and obtained a prison job. He would talk about what kind of future he wanted and about his past. However, he continued to relate with others in the same intimidating way. I did not realize until later that David was improving his behavior only because he was trying to be what he thought I wanted.

After several months of treatment, David decided that his problems would be solved if I would become his girlfriend. We talked at great length about this but nothing I said to discourage him appeared to have an impact. He began to talk about past sexual encounters in graphic detail. When I set a limit with him about this, David began to try to engage me in arguments. At one point during this time, he said that if he could not succeed at sexually arousing me, the next best thing he could do was to piss me off.

It was at this point in the treatment that I began to consider that David had predominately psychopathic traits. He was going through the motions of therapy and making what appeared to be progress. However, I could not attach to him. I never sensed that we engaged. As the therapy progressed, it became clearer that I was not another person to David—I was only someone to be used.

When David realized that a sexual relationship between us was not going to happen, he began to threaten to kill me. I removed him from my caseload and alerted custodial staff. We were able to meet many months later with other staff present. I apologized for not providing him with proper treatment. He apologized for the threats and he posed no further problems to me.

A Hidden Minority

Establishing a new identity based on sobriety and prosocial behavior is an overwhelming endeavor. In order to achieve successful secondary desistance and identity change, new and tenuously held skills and capacities must be employed. Former friends and acquaintances associated with the criminal and drug-addicted subcultures have to be disavowed. It is also likely that new intimate relationships have to be forged. The replacement of a social network is an alienating and lonely experience, making the effects of positive prosocial relationships even more pronounced.

During this transition, desisters become a hidden minority (Rubin & Babbie, 2008). Once ex-offenders are integrated into the community with stable housing and an adequate, steady income, they can "disappear." They are no longer visible to their previous subculture nor are they recognized by the larger community. As necessary as these changes may be, they can leave desisters with a split mental life, an "ongoing tension with their sense of self" (Aresti et al., 2010, p. 182).

On the one hand, the successful desister has his new life and identity. It is quite possible that the people he interacts with in this realm know nothing about his previous life. On the other hand, especially during periods of stress and frustration, the desister maintains an ongoing memory of his former lifestyle. Not all dissociated self-states are processed through therapy. Some that represent old behaviors endure during this tenuous time, increasing the risk of recidivism. As Mark, with over 10 years of sobriety and prosocial behavior, so wisely stated, "Damn, I still have a long way to go. You know what I mean? I don't do a lot of things but I haven't forgotten how to do what I used to do." Therapy can play an important role in helping clients explore the more subtle demands of long-term identity integration, providing support during this difficult phase of mental bifurcation.

Clinical Case Example

Jerry was a 55-year-old divorced white male at the time he was referred for outpatient therapy by his original therapist who had treated him during his incarceration. She had run into him at the grocery store where they both worship. He was complaining of increasing agitation, depression, and urges to use. Jerry had served time in prison for drug-related crimes, had attended a treatment-based halfway house, and had been sober and crime-free for many years. However, the experience of middle age was challenging his sense of self.

Obsessed by the fact that he was gaining weight, Jerry felt that his appearance was deteriorating. He described a recent break up with a girlfriend who had taken advantage of him financially. He was enraged with her and enraged with himself for remaining attached to her. He was also frustrated with his career path. Although Jerry qualified to apply to the court to have his record sealed (so that potential employers would not be able to see it), he had not pursued this avenue. When I asked why not, he said he was too busy.

Jerry began using online dating sites to meet women. He was careful to tell me that he was only pursuing women close to his own age but he also described placing significant pressure on them to have sex on the first date. He said dismissively that otherwise, the date was not worth it. Jerry reported no desire to rape the women he dated. He said if they were not interesting in complying, he simply would not see them again. This scenario occurred several times during our short treatment episode. He was dating multiple women, many of them only for one date.

Although Jerry successfully completed his previous treatment, it seemed to me that he never accepted responsibility for the damage he caused others. Jerry was humiliated by his past criminal behavior; he had not integrated what he had done into his current sense of self. His distress was evidenced by his avoidance of the court's record-sealing process.

Jerry was also unable to engage fully in intimate relationships. As he aged, this deficit created further feelings of humiliation, loss, and rage. And his choice of compulsive sexual behavior to replace his previous addictions caused further narcissistic assaults as these relationships inevitably failed. Jerry had substantial insight about his emotional condition but was without the skills to tolerate it or work through his deficits. The reflective processes and coping skills which comprise the capacity for internal conflict and personal agency appeared to be absent.

I felt inadequate when I met with Jerry. His pressured speech and presentation made me feel anxious. I was having a difficult time finding something about him to like. I felt that he could sense my struggle which increased his humiliation. Despite my efforts, I was unable to engage with him. We met for three sessions during which we discussed his current difficulties. Then Jerry dropped out. I later discovered another factor which explained his lack of engagement. The insurance claims I submitted for these sessions were denied. Jerry had lied about having health insurance; his coverage had expired. Although Jerry had stopped the most overt of his antisocial behaviors, he had never achieved full identity change and secondary desistance.

Meaning Making

Meaning making is the crowning achievement of all therapeutic work. It renders mental processes understandable and assigns coherence to the events and relationships that populate one's life. To make meaning of one's life confers a sense of purpose and answers the question, 'why am I here?' Internal conflict begins the process of meaning making (Holmes, 2011) as it brings about the ability for self-reflection. However, the capacity to make meaning of one's life fully forms only after personal agency has been established and identity secured. Meaning making transcends seeing oneself differently. It expands perspective from seeing oneself as a solitary individual to seeing oneself within the context of one's life.

The capacity for meaning making takes on special significance when one's life has been rife with suffering. Goldberg and Crespo (2003) stated that without a sense of personal meaning with which to overcome suffering, many "remain in a disabled and anguished state" (p. 85). Yet trying to make sense of how a loved one could ignore, neglect, hurt, or abuse is one of the most difficult aspects of the healing process.

Witnessing is a crucial mechanism in making meaning out of suffering. Viewing the process from a constructivist and relational stance, Goldberg and Crespo (2003) explained that pain does not become suffering until it is translated into a category of meaning conveyed by others' perspectives and perceptions, "a learned process that is transmitted to us interpersonally" (p. 87). In a parallel manner, they also believe that the transcendence of suffering is created within an interpersonal context. The sufferer must be helped to "define himself to us as he intends" (p. 88).

Guilt and Blame

Causing suffering further complicates the task. The moral development achieved during identity change induces a painful level of introspection.

The questions asked of oneself expand from "Why am I here?" to include others relating to abuse or neglect such as "How can this behavior be explained to myself and others?" and "How can I live with and make sense of what I did, especially after hurting or killing a loved one?" In order to answer these questions, those who have hurt others through their actions must accept responsibility for those actions and experience guilt.

The acceptance of responsibility for previous harmful behavior is a crucial task of treatment with substance abusers and offenders. Without awareness of one's impact on others, the new identity formed will be incapable of genuine intimacy. As in Jerry's case example, the capacity to engage in emotional vulnerability as well as to tolerate and accept others' will not fully form. Without acknowledgment of past abusive behavior, the client will remain at risk of regression to hurtful acts.

During successful therapy, the nature and quality of blame undergoes a profound transformation. Early in treatment, those engaging in substance abuse and offending behavior project blame to others. Nothing is their fault; others either caused or deserved their bad behavior. Through the attachment and identification processes, clients undergo a shift in how they view themselves and others. They learn through their experience in therapy the meaning of being treated with dignity and respect as well as understanding the level of disrespect with which they had previously treated others. Only when clients gain control of their behavior through the capacity for internal conflict and personal agency can they genuinely accept responsibility for their choices and comprehend and accept others' blame. True guilt and remorse are indicators of a healthy personality structure.

As with the process that translates an individual's pain into an understood sense of suffering, the witness who shares his or her understanding and perspective with the abuser translates the pain caused to others into an understanding of their suffering. This level of awareness requires an exploration of the impact of the damage including the abuser's past mental states and difficulties which precipitated the behaviors as well as how the actions impacted others at the individual, familial, community, and societal levels.

Yet this function must be incorporated carefully into therapeutic work in order avoid overwhelming the client by the negative affect generated during the exploration of causing harm, accepting responsibility, assigning blame to the self, and becoming cognizant of the damage done to others, particularly because these meanings will be constructed as the result of the therapist's perspective. Otherwise, it is easy for desisters with a newly formed and shaky sense of self to regress to blaming others or negative acting out behavior. Several techniques can enhance support for the client's new identity during this process.

It is important for the therapist to remind the client of the purpose of the examination: to find meaning, strengthen one's sense of self, and help internalize ways to avoid harmful behavior in the future. Mitchell (1993) stated that forgiveness for aggressive self-states and behavior involves reparation toward real others, internal objects, and the self. It may be helpful to define healthy guilt and self-blame for the client. Functional guilt and self-blame serve both to prevent behavior that has been labeled as wrong and to stop behavior that is in process once determined to be wrong. On the contrary, dysfunctional guilt causes overwhelming self-hatred that must be escaped by external coping mechanisms. It does not address the actions which initiated it nor will it affect ongoing behavior. These explanations serve to remind the client of the therapeutic attachment despite the therapist's feedback about the client's destructive behavior.

Other support systems can be utilized as well. The 12 Step programs' disease model incorporates the acceptance of blame for addiction-based behavior without self-hatred. As Lee learned in the program, he was not in his right mind when drinking. By following their mandates, organized religious or spiritual practice can offer a path to self-forgiveness about damage and hurt caused to loved ones. If clients are not attending 12 Step or worship services, the therapist can explain how these perspectives support a self-affirming acknowledgment of guilt.

The process of client meaning making will have a profound effect upon therapists as well. The therapist will have experienced an evolution of attitudes about his or her client's bad behavior. In the beginning, it is difficult to tolerate the client's demanding and self-centered behavior while the abuse of others continues with impunity. The attachment process along with the client's improving behavior softens the therapist's view of his or her client. Processing dissociated self-states through ruptures and enactment, co-creating the capacities for internal conflict and personal agency, and sharing in another's transformation from being an abuser of self and others to a sober and thoughtful person are powerful mechanisms through which the therapist can then view the destructive behavior. Once client and therapist together explore the damage done to others, they can proceed to gain an understanding and make meaning of this life in which suffering was both experienced and created. The therapist may also undergo shifts in his or her states of aggression, self-blame, and capacity for self-forgiveness as a result of this process.

The Role of Narratives

Meaning making is developed through the creation of a self-narrative, a story about how the seemingly random environments and situations transpiring over time came together to produce a coherent thread representing this person in the here and now. Our brains are configured to interpret salient events and experiences into a narrative which produces "a meaning from lived experience" (Forrest, 2013, p. 17). This story must be told to another in order for it to have form and cohesion. In the case of now sober and prosocial clients, their story can be told through the co-constructed nature of the therapy.

As personal agency evolves into meaning making, the task of therapy becomes to produce a consistent and shared narrative (Bragin, 2010) with which to understand and make sense of the client's life events and life changes. 12 Step programs provide another means with which to develop a prosocial self-narrative. Their testimonials provide a public forum in which members can craft and tell their stories. Meaning making can also be included in the termination process as looking back and seeing the course and progress of therapy strengthens and reinforces the internalization and narrative processes.

Meaning making when there is a history of hurting or abusing others often produces the motivation to make amends. Half of the study respondents volunteered in soup kitchens, shelters, and within their 12 Step programs. Several worked within the field of social services and several more discussed their plans to become substance abuse counselors. In doing so, clients experience another aspect of a healthy life: the ability to set and achieve goals for the purpose of personal growth. Helping others adds a chapter to one's self-narrative as it reinforces prosocial identity.

Clinical Case Example

Henry was a 40-year-old married white male who had been released from prison 3 years before meeting with me for therapy. He had served a 12-year sentence for manslaughter. Mandated to outpatient mental health counseling by his parole officer due to relapses with narcotics, Henry had completed detox and was struggling to remain sober. He desperately wanted to reestablish relationships with his two children, aged 21 and 18. They were struggling with their own addictions and he wanted to help them avoid the life course he had followed.

Henry attended AA and had received some counseling while incarcerated. A statement made in one of his group meetings had stayed with him: Nothing changes if nothing changes. He said at first he found the saying obnoxious and irritating, more so because he could not get it out of his head. As we talked about it, he realized that he did not understand it but that it also had something important to tell him about the nature of change.

We talked about the concept of personal agency. I explained that creating conditions in his life in which others were forced to make decisions for him guaranteed that the actions taken would not be to his liking. Henry began to learn and practice coping skills and strategies that enabled him to remain sober. He met with his children and worked to establish their trust. We talked about how to provide guidance for them in a way that they could accept it, not by harsh, judgmental, and angry pronouncements but in kind, encouraging, and loving ways.

As Henry was able to help his children stabilize, he began to think about the man he had killed. He talked about his realization that the crime he committed deprived his victim of being able to do exactly what Henry was doing. With shock, Henry said that his victim never got to see his children grow up nor could he help them transition to adulthood.

We talked about how to manage the guilt this realization brought. Since Henry was active in NA and was working on his steps, he wanted to be able to make amends. He talked with his sponsor and with me about the difficulty of this task because making amends to the family of his victim was not appropriate. In lieu of making direct amends, Henry committed to remaining active in the 12 Step community and living a crime- and substance-free life. He helped others in early recovery by providing transportation to meetings and becoming a sponsor. He also decided to volunteer to talk to adolescents and young adults at risk of drug abuse to help them avoid the life that he had chosen. His ongoing commitment to his sobriety became the avenue with which he made amends for his past destructive behavior. It also helped him to make sense of the direction his life had taken.

Conclusion

The process of relationally based therapy with substance abusers and offenders is complicated and demanding. When the client's life is crisis-based and filled with danger, it is difficult to create and maintain the core features of attachment, care, concern, emotional warmth, and safety. Once treatment is established, attachment between therapist and client is continually challenged by treatment ruptures and enactments and the ongoing processes of witnessing and containment. Attempts to maintain therapeutic holding throughout this turmoil can feel as if one is riding a deranged rollercoaster—desperately holding on while it careens on old and rusted tracks, with jarring ups and downs at dangerous speeds and at constant risk of derailment.

Yet, successful relationally based treatment offers many benefits to both client and therapist. Due to the mutual nature of the therapeutic relationship, both individuals grow and gain capacities as the therapy progresses. Through the turmoil and chaos, the client gains a decision-making process integrated among his or her major self-states and learns to manage feeling states effectively and without reliance on substances. These capacities are based on proficiencies in affect management, introspection, and insight as well as internalized cognitive skills gained from two types of identification: knowledge directly provided by the therapist and the client's internalizing the therapist's affective and cognitive capabilities through the course of the work. Further capacities for a cohesive sense of self and emotional intimacy in interpersonal relationships promote the ability to maintain a prosocial lifestyle. Client and therapist co-create a narrative with which the client can make sense of his or her transition from substance abuse and criminal behavior to becoming a sober, crime-free, thoughtful, and caring member of the community with much to offer others.

However, given the many challenges to treatment based on the deficits inherent in clients, therapists, and service delivery systems, success in treatment rarely occurs as a result of one long-term episode of individual treatment as described in this chapter. The many intricate mechanisms of relational therapy must be maintained in order to promote and facilitate desistance yet multiple factors conspire to defeat this task. The following chapter is devoted to applying relational concepts to real world scenarios: the short-term, CBT-based, group modalities most commonly offered offenders by the publicly funded agencies from which they seek help.

References

Altman, N. (2005). Psychoanalysis and the urban poor. In L. Aron & A. Harris (Eds.), *Relational psychoanalysis: Volume 2 innovation and expansion*. Hillsdale, NJ: Analytic Press.

American Psychiatric Association. (2013). *Diagnostic and statistical manual of mental disorders* (5th ed.). Washington, DC/London: Author.

Aresti, A., Eatough, V., & Brooks-Gordon, B. (2010). Doing time after time: An interpretive phenomenological analysis of reformed ex-prisoners' experiences of self change, identity and career opportunities. *Psychology, Crime & Law, 16*, 169–190.

Bach, S. (2006). *Getting from here to there: Analytic love, analytic process*. Hillsdale, NJ: Analytic Press.

Bass, A. (2003). "E" Enactments in psychoanalysis: Another medium, another message. *Psychoanalytic Dialogues, 13*, 657–675.

Bass, A. (2007). When the frame doesn't fit the picture. *Psychoanalytic Dialogues, 17*, 1–27.

Benjamin, J. (2009). Psychoanalytic controversies: A relational psychoanalysis perspective on the necessity of acknowledging failure in order to restore the facilitating and containing features of the intersubjective relationship (the shared third). *International Journal of Psychoanalysis, 90*, 441–450.

Benjamin, J. (2010). Where's the gap and what's the difference? The relational view of intersubjectivity, multiple selves, and enactments. *Contemporary Psychoanalysis, 46*, 112–119.

Berenguer, J. (2007). The effect of empathy in proenvironmental attitudes and behaviors. *Environment & Behavior, 39*, 269–283.

Bion, W. R. (1967). *Second thoughts*. London: Karnac.

Boston Change Process Study Group. (2013). Enactment and the emergence of new relational organization. *Journal of the American Psychoanalytic Association, 61*, 727–749.

Bragin, M. (2010). Can anyone here know who I am? Co-constructing meaningful narratives with combat veterans. *Clinical Social Work Journal, 38*, 316–326.

Bromberg, P. M. (1998). *Standing in the spaces: Essays on clinical process, trauma, & dissociation*. Hillsdale, NJ/London: Analytic Press.

Davies, J. M., & Frawley, M. G. (1994). *Treating the adult survivor of childhood sexual abuse: A psychoanalytic perspective*. New York: Basic Books.

Farber, B. A., & Lane, J. S. (2001). Positive regard. *Psychotherapy: Theory, Research, Practice, Training, 38*, 390–395.

Fonagy, P. (2001). *Attachment theory and psychoanalysis*. New York: Other Press.

Fonagy, P., Roth, A., & Higgitt, A. (2005). Psychodynamic psychotherapies: Evidence-based practice and clinical wisdom. *Bulletin of the Menninger Clinic, 69*, 1–58.

Forrest, K. (2013). *Moments, attachment and formations of selfhood: Dancing with now*. Basingstoke: Palgrave Macmillan.

Frankel, J. (2002). Exploring Ferenczi's concept of identification with the aggressor: Its role in trauma, everyday life, and the therapeutic relationship. *Psychoanalytic Dialogues, 12*, 101–139.

Gabbard, G. O., & Westen, D. (2003). Rethinking therapeutic action. *International Journal of Psycho-Analysis, 83*, 823–841.

Gaztambide, D. J. (2012). Psychotherapy for the people. *Contemporary Psychoanalysis, 48*, 141–165.

Goldberg, C., & Crespo, V. (2003). Suffering and personal agency. *International Journal of Psychotherapy, 8*, 85–93.

Harris, A. E. (2010). The relational tradition: Landscape and canon. *Journal of the American Psychoanalytic Association, 59*, 701–735.

Holmes, J. (2011). Donnel Stern and relational psychoanalysis. *British Journal of Psychotherapy, 27*, 305–315.

Iqbal, A. (2015). The ethical considerations of psychologists working with trauma: Is there a risk of vicarious traumatization? *Counseling Psychology Review, 30*, 44–51.

Lyons-Ruth, K. (2005). The two-person unconscious: Intersubjective dialogue, enactive relational representation, and the emergence of new forms of relational organization. In L. Aron & A. Harris (Eds.), *Relational psychoanalysis: Volume 2 innovation and expansion* (pp. 311–352). Hillsdale, NJ/London: Analytic Press.

Miller, W. R., & Rollnick, S. (2002). *Motivational interviewing: Preparing people for change* (5th ed.). New York/London: The Guilford Press.

Mitchell, S. A. (1993). Aggression and the endangered self. *Psychoanalytic Quarterly, 62*, 351–382.

Modell, A. H. (1991). The therapeutic relationship as a paradoxical experience. *Psychoanalytic Dialogues, 1*, 13–28.

Rothschild, D. (2010). Partners in treatment: Relational psychoanalysis and harm reduction therapy. *Journal of Clinical Psychology: In Session, 66*, 136–149.

Rubin, A., & Babbie, E. R. (2008). *Research methods for social work* (6th ed.). Belmont, CA: Thompson.

Russell, P. L. (2006a). On waiting for the right time. *Smith College Studies in Social Work, 76*, 99–104.

Russell, P. L. (2006b). The compulsion to repeat. *Smith College Studies in Social Work, 76*, 33–49.

Safran, J. D., & Kraus, J. (2014). Alliance ruptures, impasses and enactments: A relational perspective. *Psychotherapy, 51*, 381–387.

Skeem, J. L., Eno Louden, J., Polaschek, D., & Camp, J. (2007). Assessing relationship quality in mandated community treatment: Blending care with control. *Psychological Assessment, 19*, 397–410.

Slochower, J. (2005). Holding: Something old and something new. In L. Aron & A. Harris (Eds.), *Relational psychoanalysis: Volume 2 innovation and expansion* (pp. 29–50). Hillsdale, NJ/London: Analytic Press.

Snyder, C. R. (2002). Hope theory: Rainbows in the mind. *Psychological Inquiry, 13*, 249–275.

Stern, D. B. (2010). Partners in thought: Working with unformulated experience, dissociation, and enactment. In D. B. Stern (Ed.), *Psychoanalysis in a new key* (Vol. 12). New York/London: Routledge.

Taylor, P. J., McMurran, M., & Reiss, D. (2007). Coherence and complexity: Developing strategies for prevention and remediation of harm when major mental disorders, substance misuse and offending co-occur. *Criminal Behavior and Mental Health, 17*, 193–196.

Williams, A. M., Helm, H. M., & Clemens, E. V. (2012). The effect of childhood trauma, personal wellness, supervisory working alliance, and organizational factors on vicarious traumatization. *Journal of Mental Health Counseling, 34*, 133–153.

Winnicott, D. W. (1958). *Collected papers: Through pediatrics to psychoanalysis.* New York: Basic Books.

7

Relational Therapy and the "Real World"

Abstract The final chapter grapples with the application of relational practice theory to "real world" situations. Current treatment environments are described in terms of the pressures and constraints that prevent the long-term relationally based individual therapy model that psychodynamic theory espouses. Types of treatment typically offered in publicly funded agencies that provide the care for substance abusers and offender are discussed. Methods of integrating relationally based concepts and interventions in short-term and long-term group work with clients in primary desistance are described. More treatment options including individual therapy are generally available for those clients in secondary desistance. The treatment issues which arise specific to this phase are explored. The chapter concludes with the author's plea for relationally informed treatment for this client population.

During the course of the interviews, study respondents described their ability to employ treatment relationships to facilitate their desistance from substance abuse and criminal behavior. Relational analytic theory was applied to understand this desistance process because it utilizes the mechanisms described by respondents to provide the cognitive and

© The Editor(s) (if applicable) and The Author(s) 2016

D.H. Benveniste, *Changing Substance Abuse and Criminal Behavior Through Therapeutic Relationships*, DOI 10.1057/978-1-137-53039-4_7

affective skills needed to renounce these behaviors. However, relational analytic theory is not often applied to working with clients with severe disorders and who obtain their treatment from publicly funded and private non-profit agencies. The practice theory is based on a long-term individual therapy model.

Unfortunately, many aspects of the current treatment climate prevent the use of this type of practice. Sociopaths are routinely considered unamenable to individual therapy because they are viewed as being incapable of therapeutic engagement or remorse. Substance abusers are known for their crisis-oriented lifestyle and manipulation of others for their own ends. Many in the mental health field consider both of these client groups to be unworkable through any means. Yet, even if they are considered able to benefit from treatment, the life situations and problems these groups bring create ongoing management crises which can easily scuttle any attempts at treatment. Facilities that offer services to these client populations encounter their own obstacles as well.

Societal Marginalization and Access to Treatment

Poverty and societal marginalization place significant demands on the treatment endeavor both in terms of the clients and the agencies which provide their care. Poor and disempowered clients are less likely to have the means and resources to seek their own treatment, more likely to be involved with the criminal justice system, and more likely to be mandated to publicly funded facilities for their treatment. Therapists with clients mandated by state agencies have to answer to the system which mandated the client, creating additional work. Furthermore, the needs of these agencies are often at odds with clients' treatment needs. Counselors can have triple and sometimes conflicting allegiances: to their employer, the state agency mandating treatment, and lastly to the client.

Concomitantly, publicly funded and private not-for-profit counseling and mental health agencies are also marginalized, poorly funded, and mandated to provide certain types of treatment. In a state of crisis themselves, they furnish services to the most difficult and demanding clients with little public funding or support. Conservative voices in the public debate about human services wholeheartedly reject the practice of paying taxes so that criminals and drug addicts can get "free" care.

State agencies which fund treatment are under pressure to provide the most service at the least possible cost. As a result, they determine the types of treatment publicly funded facilities can offer. For example, departments of mental health and substance abuse services may mandate particular types of interventions based on the most recent research. At the unethical end of this continuum, probation and parole departments that directly fund treatment for their parolees and probationers sometimes require the treating agency to allow their officers to sit in on group therapy sessions for those mandated to counseling in order to further monitor their caseloads, upending confidentiality.

Treatment staff is overwhelmed by huge caseloads, massive amounts of paperwork, and stifling treatment protocols. Burnout is epidemic. Altman (2005) described a parallel between therapist burnout and that experienced by the poor person. He said that both are tempted to surrender and withdraw in the face of the chronic anxiety, despair, and sense of futility brought on by the client's symptoms and social situation. For the therapist, these reactions also emanate from the demands of the facility and the accompanying lack of support of its employees. For example, clinical supervision is often a victim of staffing pressures and the frenetic pace of agency work.

Treatment models for clients who offend and abuse substances reflect these negative attitudes. Despite the long-term and severe nature of these problems, interventions for the most part are offered in short-term group formats designed to minimize or eliminate relational aspects of care. CBT-based skills are taught in groups lasting between 12 and 15 weeks where the treatment is manualized. The topics are preset and the group discussion is highly structured, discouraging spontaneous and individualized interaction. Emotional dependence on the therapist and the concept of long-term supportive counseling are abhorred.

Many clinicians fear their clients becoming dependent on them, particularly those therapists who are untrained in how to understand and manage the therapeutic relationship. This training deficit causes increased pressure on the capacity of the relationship to facilitate change as the change process is so sensitive to therapeutic attachment. Yet too much or pathological dependence on the therapist can cause the therapy to stall. From a relational perspective, a therapy in which the client is too dependent on the therapist is in the thralls of an enactment of collusion. It is critical to be able to differentiate pathological dependence from healthy attachment. See the previous chapter for a discussion of the therapeutic uses of attachment, enactments, and therapist enabling.

In CBT-based group treatment, the client's internal affective world, the quality of his or her relationships with other group members, and the relationship with the group therapist are deemed insignificant as treatment issues because they are absent when formulating treatment goals (Practitioners of CBT might argue with this assertion, insisting that relational elements are integrated within their approach. However, CBT treatment goals remain behaviorally based). Some treatment programs for substance abusers and offenders are beginning to offer trauma-focused group work. Although a welcome addition, in most cases, trauma theory is integrated into a pre-existing CBT framework.

Therefore, the factors which study respondents labeled as crucial to their successful desistance, caring, trust, belief in the respondent, encouragement, never giving up on the respondent, ongoing support and reliability, and seeing something good in the respondent, those basic to relationally based treatment, are not considered intrinsically worthwhile goals. All of these elements conspire to ensure that clients who most need a long-term, individualized approach are least likely to get it. Furthermore, the mutual co-construction of relationally based therapy offers a counterpoint to the power imbalance integral to all types of therapy as well as the experience of marginalized clients when interacting with the larger society. An individualized treatment approach tailors treatment to be based on the client's unique constellation of symptoms and problems and reinforces respect for the individual. Manualized CBT-based groups, in which topics and discussion are pre-selected and imposed on clients, works to reinforce societal marginalization and disempowerment.

Yet, however necessary relationally based therapy may be, if it cannot be realized within the current treatment climate, it will remain at the sidelines of the human services field—a theoretical abstraction without practical application. The relational treatment model must be adjusted from its base as a long-term individual therapy practice so that it can be applied within these current constraints. There are several methods with which to integrate relational concepts into existing practice models at the different stages of desistance and treatment.

The most obvious difficulty in applying long-term relational concepts to short-term work is reaching the later stages of therapy. However, it seemed from respondents' narratives that their treatment experiences were cumulative. For the most part, the ten respondents who employed treatment to desist engaged in multiple attempts over the course of years. At several points, they gained important insights which they remembered, internalized, and integrated to build a self-system with enough skills and strengths to move from criminal to prosocial behavior. Therefore, each treatment attempt can be viewed both as its own complete intervention and simultaneously as having the potential to provide a lasting impact in facilitating client progression along the desistance pathway.

The Beginning Stages

In order to integrate relational theory from the start of treatment, emphasis can be placed in several areas: engagement with the client; processing of conflicts; and an initial assessment of relational style, needs, capacity for affect management, level and type of dissociation, and location in the desistance process. If treatment is individual and client-focused, it will entail crisis management. If it is a group, it will focus on cognitively based skill building. In either case, the beginning stages of treatment will be rife with conflict as clients desperately attempt to escape the repercussions of their decisions and behavior.

Clients' entrance to treatment is usually a result of a mandate from a state department such as a child service agency, through the court, during an incarceration, or as a result of conditions of parole. Hence, clients are angry, unstable, and still engaging in substance abuse and criminal behavior or in withdrawal. Many are not even contemplating a change in their lives. Clients and their counselors are harried and overwhelmed. Chaotic and fragmented treatment results.

One- or Two-Session Individual Crisis Intervention or Assessment Modalities

When the therapist has very limited time with clients, their instability, the level and intensity of their demands, and the fact that they are an unknown entity create immediate pressure on the therapeutic engagement process. It is important to maintain a therapeutic stance by trying to engage and be helpful in ways that are possible and appropriate. The most significant impact on clients, particularly those in acute crisis related to incarceration, is a warm and caring approach where the therapist attempts to see something good about the client. It is important for those in their first treatment attempts to associate kindness with treatment as this will improve the chances that they will try again. Clients often recall positive and meaningful exchanges with therapists, even those that occur within short-lived treatment episodes. Additionally, it is possible that some small level of identification could occur as a result of these exchanges.

No matter how angry or obnoxious a client's presentation may be, part of the assessment should entail imagining what he or she would look and act like fully engaged in secondary desistance. In this way, therapists can engage more easily with a recalcitrant and suspicious client. They may also be better able to formulate suggestions or advice and impart information basic to primary desistance which is based on their assessment of the client's functioning. It is unlikely that these elements of guidance will produce any immediate response. They are designed to be placed in the client's repository and employed as aids in the future when he or she is more capable of making use of them.

The quality of the therapeutic relationship may not be an articulated component of these initial interactions but it is likely the most important. Clients will more likely accept guidance in the form of direction to manage their crises or in a skill-building group if they feel that the therapist genuinely cares about them. Furthermore, clients' behavioral control is mostly likely at a minimum during some of these exchanges. Failed therapeutic engagement risks clients becoming overwhelmed by negative affect and acting out either toward others or themselves.

For example, Brother Nowapo described his struggles when he found out he was HIV+. He reported that he assaulted the doctor who informed him of his test results but was able to accept the guidance of a counselor at an AIDS task force when she referred him to an HIV sober house for treatment. He did not describe the interaction with the doctor but he said that the AIDS task force counselor took the time to explain to him that he could not continue to avoid treatment for HIV and then offered him a feasible option with which to address his health.

Clinical Case Example

Andy was a 28-year-old white male who had just been transferred to a maximum security prison to begin his 30-year sentence for two counts of manslaughter. During a drunken incident, Andy had killed his cousin and his cousin's friend. Andy had requested to be seen at the Mental Health Department and explained his history of alcoholism, depression, and suicide attempts. I arranged for an emergency psychiatric appointment the following day but it did not seem to me that Andy was going to make it through the night without trying to kill himself.

I could have placed Andy on a suicide watch; however, I believed that the humiliating and intrusive nature of this intervention would only increase his suicidal urges. Two things I knew at that point led me to consider an alternative. Andy mentioned how important his treatment at the local jail had been to him in terms of coping with his incarceration and the sentencing process. I also knew that he was a veteran and therefore was used to living within an austere structure of a large bureaucracy. I believed that adjusting to his new location and status as a convicted inmate was going to be more helpful to him than undergoing the further disruption a suicide watch would entail.

Andy said he thought he would be okay if he could just get some medication to help him sleep through the night. The only way for him to be started on medication without having first seen the psychiatrist would be for me to walk him to the medical unit and request Benadryl for him for sleep, which I did. I also offered him membership in the lifers' group that a colleague and I co-facilitated. He eagerly agreed. Andy survived the night, saw the psychiatrist the following day, and successfully adjusted to his prison term.

During the time he was incarcerated at this prison, Andy attended group and individual therapy faithfully as well as AA and NA meetings. He was a model inmate and completed his associate degree while there. He sponsored other inmates through the 12 Step programs and committed himself to maintaining a sober lifestyle.

Several years later, as his transfer was approaching, Andy talked in the lifers' group about the most important event in his life that redirected him to the right path. I was stunned to hear him say that it was the day I walked him to the medical unit. He said the medication was incidental in that Benadryl would not be much of a treatment for insomnia given his distress and the noise level of the cellblock. What was so important to him about the intervention was that I had gone way out of my way to help him. He said that through my eyes, he could see that despite his crimes, he was a worthwhile person who should not kill himself for what he had done.

Short-Term Group Work During Primary Desistance

Short-term work with substance abusers and offenders can take place in a detox unit, an outpatient clinic for mental health or substance abuse, a hospital, or in a prison. If the treatment consists of more than one or two meetings for crisis intervention or assessment purposes, therapists would most likely be following specific CBT-based treatment protocols. Relationally, it would be important to focus on therapeutic attachment and the process of identification. Any interpersonal conflicts within the group can be processed with an eye toward the capacity for internal conflict and aspects of personal agency. The therapist can make an internal assessment of the client's phase of desistance, needs, capacity for affect management, and level and type of dissociation.

Prochaska's Transtheoretical Model of the Stages of Change (Prochaska et al., 1994) can be a useful framework to apply to determine the client's phase of desistance. The Stages of Change continuum includes precontemplation, not thinking about change; contemplation, serious consideration of change; preparation, which includes practice behaviors; action, where negative behaviors stop; and maintenance, defined as continued change. The first two levels, precontemplation and contemplation, do not apply to the desistance process as clients have not yet made the decision to change. The preparation phase which includes practice behaviors corresponds to primary desistance while action and maintenance apply to secondary desistance.

In any given short-term group, clients' motivational levels will span the full range of the change continuum. At this point, it will be difficult if not impossible to differentiate which clients are just beginning their desistance processes versus those who are not at all contemplating changing their lifestyle. Some who appear eagerly invested in change are only seeking to avoid legal consequences of their behavior. Others who present as surly and oppositional may actually be near or at the preparation phase and primary desistance.

Since each treatment episode typically does not last long enough to make a full assessment of the motivation level of clients near or at early desistance, it is most helpful to assume their engagement in the primary desistance process. There is no harm in perceiving everyone as treatment-ready. At worst, there will be clients in the group who think the therapist is easily manipulated but for those who are ready, the stance will improve the chances for therapeutic engagement. If the therapist assumes that no one is ready, those who are will be put off by this negative judgment.

During these treatment episodes, therapists can provide encouragement and explain the fragmented nature of the treatment system. To reduce a sense of failure clients may feel due to these multiple attempts, therapists can explain that they will most likely have to engage in multiple treatments in multiple formats as a result of this system. They can also suggest that in order to make the most use of their treatment, clients will need to listen for what is most important to them and accumulate those pieces of wisdom over time and attempts. Therapists can reassure clients that these diverse pieces of information will form into a cohesive whole when the client is ready to implement a change. These suggestions are not a product of relational theory. Anyone with any type of training can point out this process to clients in an encouraging manner. What is specific to relational theory is that one of the goals of these interventions is to facilitate identification with the therapist; for the client to integrate these ideas as representing the prosocial person who shared them.

Several study respondents mentioned therapeutic experiences as critical even though they had occurred years before they entered into secondary desistance. Jay's recollection of a group therapy session, in which the group leader told him that drugs were not as much of a problem for him as was chronic incarceration, had occurred many years prior to the study interview. It was a therapeutic turning point for him. He realized that prior to that point he had been misdirecting his efforts. When Jay shared this recollection, he described the therapist in detail: how she carried his record in her arms, how she entered the room and sat down. He remembered how she stopped the process of the group to point this out to him. The piece of information was notable but the feeling of being important to that therapist was equally salient. This episode became an important part of the self-narrative of Jay's new identity which emerged many years later.

E talked about the revelation gained from his sponsor that his mother had been doing the best she could. He said his years of anger at her immediately dissipated and that he was able to change the nature of his relationship with her as a result of that piece of wisdom from his sponsor. The intervention had occurred years prior to the research interview in which he shared it with me. It came at the right moment so that E could significantly expand his relational capacities.

Ace was able to make use of a negative treatment experience to access another type of resource. He described his first treatment encounter as a detox in a private for-profit hospital. He found the program to be administered by an uninterested and uninvested staff. As a result of this relational void, he realized that spiritual guidance was crucial to him. After completing the program, Ace began attending church regularly which facilitated a reunion with his sister and her family. These important bits of information and relational capacities gleaned along the way ultimately formed a desistance plan for each of these respondents.

Integrating Relational Concepts into Longer Term Group Therapy

The relational framework can be applied to time-limited CBT-based group work although this is not an easy task. These groups generally are focused on a particular aspect of addiction or criminal behavior or on a skill set such as relapse prevention. But if clients are permitted to share their stories, the therapist can provide a witnessing function as well as role model it for other group members. Aspects of addiction or criminal behavior can be thought about and spoken about as emanating from self-states that seem to take over. These selves can be described and the transition from one to another can be explored.

If clients are permitted to interact with each other during group sessions, the relational stance can be used as a framework to understand therapeutic exchanges. The group therapist would be able to observe and assess areas of client functioning including level and type of dissociation. Warmth, caring, and respect can be reinforced as the expected tone of interactions. Aspects of identification can be explained without necessarily resorting to relational terminology. For example, therapists can talk about the importance of role models in attaining sobriety.

It is more difficult for ruptures or enactments to be managed within a group format due to the multitude of people and factors involved. Clients may reenact traumatic episodes by projecting to other group members and not to the therapist. In this case, a group member is being targeted which may trigger his or her own past abuse history. The remaining group members also experience these episodes, causing additional distress and possibly dissociated self-states.

Safety of the clients must be prioritized before any processing of the disruption can occur. The acting out client may abruptly leave the group meeting and not return to treatment or the group therapist may determine that his or her continued presence is too destabilizing to the group for this group member to remain. If these events do not occur, then the therapist can halt the progression of group discussion to discuss what occurred. If it is an enactment and the therapist is paralyzed and unable to respond, he or she can consult with the clinical supervisor after the group and bring up the episode at the next meeting. The concepts of dissociated self-states and reenacted trauma can be introduced as a means to process the disruption. Some witnessing can occur during the processing.

Without enactment and its resolution occurring between therapist and client, it will be far more difficult for clients to attain the capacity for internal conflict and the beginnings of personal agency through the relationship with the group therapist. However, the influence of other group members can compensate and help bring these capabilities about. Group members can confront each other about poor decision-making and bad behavior in a way that therapists cannot. It is possible that hearing about sober and prosocial behavior from others engaged in the same struggle can produce some aspects of internal conflict and personal agency. Certainly, group members can form identifications with each other so that they internalize and integrate each other's strengths and skills.

Lastly, if 12 Step programs are available, clients should be encouraged to attend. Although most of the discussion on the benefits of AA/NA meetings focuses on their cognitive aspects and medical/religious structure, it is important to point out to clients their relational aspects. 12 Step programs recognize the lifelong struggle that addiction imposes and provide ongoing support through meetings and sponsorships. Additionally, the testimonials and structured responses to those who speak at meetings teach members basic interpersonal skills such as listening and not interrupting when others speak to which they may have never before been exposed. The relational aspects of 12 Step programs can compensate to some degree for the lack of relational focus in formal treatment.

Partial Hospitalization or Day Treatment Programs

Partial hospitalization programs run by non-profit or for-profit hospitals offer an important alternative to outpatient treatment, particularly at the beginning of the desistance process. By providing a more comprehensive program to their clients including various types of groups and some individual and family therapy, they can address multiple areas of functioning at several intervention levels. Unfortunately, both public and insurance-based funding limit the authorization for this treatment generally to several weeks, reducing its potential. These programs would make good test sites if relationally based therapy were to be offered.

Residential Treatment/Sober Houses

Although some residential treatment models are extremely short term, others permit residents to remain for 6–12 months. However, most do not provide treatment at the facility and so clients would find themselves in the same situation with repeating episodes of short term treatment. Some support and identification can take place within the program among the residents. Dee talked about the importance to him of the older residents at his sober house and the sense of belonging they extended to him.

Treatment for Clients Approaching or in Secondary Desistance

Most clients who are functioning successfully in the prosocial community have private insurance and can access private individual therapy. In many states, however, insurance companies restrict the authorization of outpatient visits so that even within an individual therapy modality, treatment episodes may be time limited. Furthermore, therapists in private practice may lack the skill set to treat these problems, thereby either providing inadequate care or refusing to treat the client at all.

For those therapists with experience and a comfort level treating clients with offending and substance abuse histories, it should be easier to determine the phase of desistance of those further along in the change process. These clients would describe multiple past treatment attempts as well as previous periods of sobriety. They should show an ability to talk about their efforts to stop and what went wrong with each of them. They should evidence the capacity for internal conflict by describing contradictory aspects of themselves rather than blaming others for their recidivism.

Clients in full secondary desistance should not find themselves in short-term treatment unless they have relapsed, indicating that the identity change process necessary for secondary desistance had not yet fully formed. In this case, the most effective focus for treatment would be to help the client identify what pieces were missing that would have enabled continued sobriety. Relationally, it would be important to listen for indicators of deficits in personal agency and identity formation. The case of Jerry in the previous chapter presented an example of a client who had not yet reached secondary desistance despite years of sobriety. Had I been able to engage with him, we would have needed to address his shaky sense of identity and the substitute addiction which was eroding his capacity for personal agency.

Clients who have achieved full secondary desistance with a prosocial identity intact will also most likely be able to access private individual therapy. It would be important to determine the precipitant causing these clients to return; what had occurred that had threatened their stability. Despite the length of an individual's secondary desistance, he or she remains at some level of risk of recidivism due to the ongoing challenges in maintaining a prosocial identity.

Therapists need to be sensitive to how alienating it can feel when the barrier between these two worlds develops cracks. Those who can attend to the ongoing struggles that ex-offenders experience in their secondary desistance processes will be able to provide encouragement, advocacy, and guidance about how to approach the different types of challenges and obstacles that appear at the more successful levels of life. Therapeutic work on meaning making may have been previously lacking. Helping the client to take stock of his or her desistance path and make sense of the current crisis from that perspective will assist in stabilization efforts.

Clinical Case Example

Tim was a 58-year-old married African-American man with two grown children from a previous marriage. Similar to the study respondents, he described a tumultuous upbringing by drug-addicted parents who were in and out of his life. He lived in several foster homes and began using alcohol and heroin at a young age. Tim had two brief incarcerations during his 20s and utilized treatment well to change his lifestyle and give up his addictions. He continued to attend 12 Step programs over the next decades and slowly built his life into something of which he was proud.

Tim requested treatment because of marital problems. He had been married to his second wife for 10 years and in a relationship that was challenged by their personality differences and emotional restrictedness. We did some couples therapy in which they were able to practice listening to each other and learned to address each other's concerns. As their relationship stabilized, Tim began to bring up his impending retirement from a job that despite his addictions and incarcerations, he had managed to keep since his 20s. He said he was beginning to experience urges to use and leave his wife so that he could "run free."

Although he did not realize it, Tim's job had been a major stabilizing force in his being able to desist. We talked about his efforts to maintain the job throughout the years and how valued he felt when his employer rehired him after his incarcerations. As a result, he had prioritized his employment as most important which helped him in his struggle to avoid drugs and alcohol. Now he was about to lose this structure.

Successful retirement was not something Tim had ever contemplated. No one he knew as a youngster or as an addict had ever maintained a skilled job long enough to access retirement benefits. Despite his success, part of Tim's sense of self still identified as an addict, someone who did not deserve his current situation. The status change to successful retiree threatened Tim's identity. He was uncomfortable with the idea of joining the retired community. We spent session time discussing issues related to internal conflict as he was experiencing urges to use, his identity as a prosocial community member who was about to retire, and meaning making as Tim did not realize his level of emotional attachment to his employment and employer.

As we explored his employer functioning in many ways as the stable and supportive parental figure that Tim had missed in his early life, Tim began to experience grief he had not before consciously felt. And with this came a treatment rupture. Tim began telling me of his plans to drain his retirement accounts without telling his wife and to purchase run-down properties in order to "flip" them. He became morally outraged when I questioned this plan, perceiving my response as a lack of trust in his money management skills.

Because we had done couples work as part of his treatment, this argument was familiar to me. It was one in which Tim often had engaged his wife when they were struggling. I asked why we were having this fight. He tried a few more times to provoke me into responding to this self by berating him as one would a child. However, I was not dissociating in response and therefore this exchange did not reach the level of an enactment.

Tim had progressed far enough in treatment that I could point out that his grief was causing dissociation; that the current self-state who was impulsively seeking to throw it all away took over because his grief about losing his employment, his previous self as a worker, and the original loss of his parents had become overwhelming. I talked about what an important achievement successful retirement is and that he had every right to be frightened. Tim started to chuckle and said he was very afraid of the status change as well as the urges he had been experiencing.

As a result, we were able to speak more freely about the impacts on Tim including all of the losses. I reassured him that although he was losing many important people and structures in his life, his treatment would continue as would his marriage. I also pointed out that in bringing this self to session, he was sparing his wife from having to reexperience it which prevented a destabilization of their relationship. Several weeks later, Tim announced that he and his wife had been talking a great deal about how to plan for both of their retirements. They decided together to purchase a second home in which to eventually retire.

Conclusion: A Plea for Relationally Informed Treatment

One of the major difficulties of using relational concepts in our CBT-based mental health treatment environment is the lack of agency support for this work. Most supervisors are not relationally or psychodynamically trained and may find these concepts alien and threatening. The solutions for this situation are inadequate. Therapists would need to read on their own, attend trainings in relational work, or hire their own clinical consultant familiar with relational and psychodynamic treatment. It can be a lonely experience.

However, even if it cannot be utilized directly, relational theory can also function as an internalized framework from which the therapist can understand clients' internal worlds and relational patterns. When ruptures and enactments occur, as they invariably will, employing a relational perspective can prepare therapists to approach and manage therapeutic conflicts in ways that not only spare the treatment but move it forward, thereby preventing countless treatment failures and premature terminations. Knowing how to manage therapeutic conflicts relationally feels empowering, improves therapists' self-esteem and sense of competence, and reduces burnout.

No matter how mentally ill or functionally disabled clients may present themselves, engagement with them from a relational perspective involves looking for meaningful ways to attach and to experience each client as a unique individual with the potential to become healthy and desist from their disabling behaviors. However, the consequences of such attachment may be significant. They include increased anxiety about clients' welfare and emotional pain if they drop out or fail at the treatment, get themselves incarcerated, or die. Furthermore, due to short-term treatment models, we do not often get to see the results of our efforts.

Yet just as often, another therapist along the way will be able to glean our previous work. At each treatment attempt, the client may be more able to engage and to articulate inner states. Representations of previous therapists' affective capacities and cognitive skills internalized through identification will be evidenced among the client's repertoire of skills and capabilities. At the end of the process, someone who had wreaked much interpersonal and societal damage is transformed into a capable and giving member of society with previously untapped relational capacities. If some of those clients choose to work in the social services, these capacities are then shared generationally, passed down from the client to his or her own clients.

Engaging with clients from a relational framework can function as a protection against other sources of burnout because it helps to prevent desensitization accrued from short-term repetitive treatments and very high caseloads. Clients begin to look and sound very similar to each other in short-term group modalities. It can be tiring to provide the same very valid and important but nevertheless repetitive CBT-based information and material. Furthermore, clients fail at their treatment attempts routinely. It is easy to become overwhelmed by despair and frustration, to expect this outcome all the time and for everyone.

When we have similar problems, despite the fact that each of us is an individual, our thoughts and behaviors can appear tediously generic. It is our personal histories, our affective internal worlds, relational capacities, and our resulting distinctive perspectives that render each of us unique. Each time we deeply engage in a relationship with another, these aspects of ourselves meld with another's to create a completely new entity, one which has never before been experienced. Different parts of ourselves are actuated as we fully engage with the other. Our character grows and develops, a creative and life-affirming process crucial to healthy functioning. The ability to engage with others and to attend to these relationships is what keeps us all emotionally alive and healthy, offering the potential of healing and strengthening us to be best able to do this very challenging and difficult work.

References

Altman, N. (2005). Psychoanalysis and the urban poor. In L. Aron & A. Harris (Eds.), *Relational psychoanalysis: Volume 2 innovation and expansion*. Hillsdale, NJ: Analytic Press.

Prochaska, J. O., Velicer, W. F., Rossi, J. S., Goldstein, M. G., Marcus, N. H., Rakowski, W., et al. (1994). Stages of change and decisional balance for 12 problem behaviors. *Health Psychology, 13*, 39–46.

Appendix: Study Rationale and Methodology

Almost all criminological attention is focused on the quantitative prediction of when and how adolescent males initiate criminal careers (Soothill et al., 2009) producing data that is limited in scope and highly compartmentalized (Curtis, 2010). A review of criminological and criminal justice research found that only approximately 6 % of published studies utilized qualitative methodology (Tewksbury, Dabney, & Copes, 2010) employing offenders' self-report.

Yet, in his text on methodological issues in the qualitative study of crime, Bernasco (2010) stated that many aspects of crime can be learned only from offenders' reports. Data related to the internal thoughts and perceptions of offenders collected via fieldwork and interviews are required in order to fully understand the factors that influence the commission of crime (Brookman, 2010; Jacques & Wright, 2010). Known as offender-based research, this method of study analyzes the accounts of offenders in their own words (Bernasco, 2010) in order to understand the processes involved in the initiation, maintenance, and desistance from criminal behavior.

Many researchers have categorized desistance as the least understood aspect of criminal behavior (Loeber et al., 2007; Maruna, 2001; Moffitt, 1993). Thoughts, feelings, perceptions, and motivations, those aspects of

© The Editor(s) (if applicable) and The Author(s) 2016

D.H. Benveniste, *Changing Substance Abuse and Criminal Behavior Through Therapeutic Relationships*, DOI 10.1057/978-1-137-53039-4

lived experience comprising internal life, are the best data by which to understand the changes of behavior and identity requisite to the desistance process. Therefore, offender-based research in the form of interviews with former offenders would best examine this phenomenon. However, of the qualitative research of offenders and former offenders reviewed for this study, none concentrated solely on adult men living in the community who had been successfully refraining from violent behavior. Although several studies addressed the role of significant relationships in the desistance process, none explored how relationships function to produce this change.

This very specific process was the subject of inquiry of this research. This interview-based study explored the psychological mechanisms in operation as the interpersonal aspects of significant relationships facilitate the process of respondents' shift in identity from criminal to law-abiding community member. It was devoted to examining the means by which affective, cognitive, and behavioral changes necessary for desistance emanate from experiencing the beneficial effects of significant relationships. The sample was composed of 11 men over the age of 25 with a history of violent behavior, residing in the community for at least 5 years after an incarceration.

This study was produced for a social work doctoral program by a seasoned clinician and explored a psychological process. The traditional criminal justice research model of quantitative comparisons of causality and prediction of crime does not suit social work values of social justice and empowerment of marginalized populations nor would it capture the workings of an internal developmental process. A departure from typical methods was necessary.

Hence, I decided to do a qualitative study interviewing men in the community who had successfully maintained prosocial behavior after a history of violent behavior. The study's methodology reflects a critical research approach that emphasizes respondents' involvement in the design and implementation of the study. The goal of such research is to "critique and challenge, to transform and empower" (Merriam & Associates, 2002, p. 327). The qualitative nature of this study gives voice to a marginalized group, one whose viewpoints and perspectives are rarely sought. Richardson (1990) describes narrative research of marginalized groups as "the textual enfranchisement of the previously disenfranchised" (p. 64).

However, the use of qualitative methods with those with a history of criminality causes a variety of difficulties, particularly related to accessing participants and procedural ethics. Despite this complexity, little is written about how to approach qualitative research with this population (Presser, 2008). It is my hope that this discussion of methodology will aid future qualitative researchers. The following topics are addressed: working definitions of variables, data sources, study design, data management and analysis, ethical concerns, trustworthiness of the data, and methodological challenges that occurred once the study was underway.

Working Definitions of Variables

Violence

This study defined violence as acts committed against people as determined by state statute and limited to those perpetrated by adult males. Any type of violent behavior, including that related to family environments, encounters with strangers, and those occurring during the commission of other offenses, met the study criteria.

Desistance

The operationalized definition of secondary desistance included: (1) self-report of a history of at least one violent offense that was adjudicated through the CJ system; and (2) self-report of a period of no incarcerations or any violent behavior for a minimum of 5 years. If during that 5-year (or longer) period, the respondent reported that he engaged in non-violent criminal activity, an assessment was made to determine if the behaviors conformed to a primary desistance process.

Significant Relationships

Consistent with the literature, significant relationships were defined as those constituting a strong attachment and close emotional ties with non-criminally involved others, including aspects of (1) care, concern, and warmth; (2) trust; (3) guidance; (4) support; and (5) a sense of belonging (Aresti, Eatough, & Brooks-Gordon, 2010; Farrall, 2004; Haggard,

Gumpert, & Grann, 2001; Hughes, 1998; Meisenhelder, 1982; Rains-Russell, 2009; Walker, 2010).

Data Sources

Data was generated solely from a semi-structured interview lasting between 60 and 90 minutes which was audio-taped and transcribed. It began with a general question to elicit the respondent's desistance narrative and included probes to elaborate information related to the role of significant relationships. A brief questionnaire about demographics followed including queries about the respondent's age, race, marital status, SES, employment, schooling, and living situation.

Study Design

Pilot Study

A pilot study was conducted in order to evaluate the interview schedule and the data collection process. The community advisor to my doctoral committee, a man who met the criteria for the study, agreed to serve as the respondent. Feedback resulted in several changes to data collection. It was my original intent to include respondents' criminal records as a data source. However, as a result of the pilot study and the committee's concerns about confidentiality and potential harm, this data collection method was abandoned. The most important conclusion I gleaned from the pilot study was that I would need to structure the interview to maintain its focus on respondents' desistance processes. The pilot study respondent spent most of the interview discussing the initiation and maintenance of his criminal career. Focused questions and probes utilized later in the interview enabled him to articulate his desistance process.

Sampling and Recruitment Procedures

Except for two, all of the researchers of qualitative studies of desistance of offenders or ex-offenders reviewed for this study obtained access to their samples through partnering with CJ agencies. However, partnering with the CJ system to obtain research respondents appeared problematic for this study for several reasons. The system imposes significant vulnerabilities on those within its purview. I believed potential respondents were likely to be less suspicious of my motives as a researcher if they were approached outside of their CJ system status. Additionally, probation or parole supervision confers structure and guidance, making it impossible to know if respondents under CJ supervision would continue to refrain from criminal activity after their discharge from parole or probation. Lastly, the study interview is focused on the transformation of respondents' identities. To utilize the criminal justice system as the recruitment method would reinforce the respondent's identity as a criminal rather than as a desister. However, desisters who are not on probation or parole become a hidden minority (Rubin & Babbie, 2008). Once they have established themselves as non-criminal members of society, they become difficult to access without the cooperation of organizations that serve them or where they are employed or volunteer their time. Therefore, I decided to partner with agencies that provided services to ex-offenders to access respondents.

Non-random, purposeful sampling means including snowball and convenience techniques were utilized. Eligible respondents were adult males over age 25 living in the community who met the study criteria specified in the Definitions section. Men who were serving parole or probation sentences at the time they contacted me about the study were excluded.

Paying respondents for their participation was important. Money is an established incentive in research with stigmatized individuals as it serves to underscore the value to the study of their participation, helping respondents "buy in" to the goals of the research (Curtis, 2010, p. 151). Respondents were paid $25 cash for their participation and a respondent who agreed to recruit others for the study was paid $10 per additional respondent found.

In January 2012, I approached two agencies in southern New England that administer programs for ex-offenders. I met with the directors of both organizations and they arranged for me to meet with staff. I provided a written letter explaining the nature of the study and recruitment flyers to be distributed at each facility. I discussed the recruitment protocol that details how to approach potential respondents. I explained the importance of not placing any undue influence on potential respondents to participate in the study and that communication from staff that is perceived as pressure will not allow for freely given consent.

I was able to access four members of my sample through the one of the organizations, including Jay, who agreed to recruit for me. He referred two clients of an HIV sober house and one client and two volunteers from a homeless shelter. One additional respondent was employed by the other agency and another self-referred when he overheard others talking about the study. I screened a total of 15 people; three did not meet the criteria and one had moved out of state before the interview could take place. The final sample consisted of 11 respondents with interviews taking place between February and April 2012.

Process of Communication with Respondents

Respondents called a phone number connected to a voice mailbox at Simmons College that instructed callers to leave their contact information. During the initial telephone communication, I described the purpose of the study and explained the procedures. A screening tool was used to determine if the potential respondent met the study criteria. Callers were informed that $25 cash would be given as an incentive. I called respondents the day before the scheduled interview to confirm the meeting.

Three interviews took place at one of the agencies, four were held at the HIV sober house, three were held at a medical clinic where most respondents received their care, and one occurred at the local public library. In consenting to be interviewed at agencies where respondents received services, they understood that their participation in the study would not be anonymous. The importance of maintaining respondent confidentiality was emphasized to staff specifically because anonymity would be impossible to establish in this circumstance. The consent form stated that results may be presented at a variety of scholarly or academic venues.

At the agency and the sober house, staff vacated the only office so I could use it to conduct the interviews. They also helped to coordinate the interview schedule to avoid conflicts with members' meetings or appointments. I reserved a conference room at the medical clinic that they generously offered at no charge. The interview at the public library took place in an area set away from where most activity was occurring. When meeting with a respondent, I introduced the study, went over the consent form, and obtained consent. I then asked for a pseudonym. Follow-up was offered including a list of resources. The cash remuneration was provided once the interview was completed.

The interview followed a semi-structured protocol and was limited to 90 minutes. In order to allow the interview to unfold and to ensure that my approach to the study did not influence respondents' answers, the interview began with more general questions and probes. Mid-way through the interview, the influence of significant relationships was introduced as an area of exploration. Following the interview, I asked the questions in the demographics questionnaire verbally and transcribed respondents' answers.

I completed a contact summary form immediately after each interview that included the date, place, and length of the interview and consisted of questions about main themes, what stood out for me, if I needed to change the interview schedule or meet with my committee about the interview, what unasked-for material did I get and why, and my feelings during the interview.

Data Management

Interviews were audio-taped on a digital tape recorder and uploaded to a password-protected computer. I transcribed five of the interviews myself. The remaining six were transcribed by an audio transcription center that signed a confidentiality agreement. I reviewed the transcribed interviews twice by comparing the audio interviews with the written transcript and utilized NVivo 9 software to do the coding and analysis.

Data Analysis

I began the analysis by coding phrases and paragraphs based on my provisional code list as determined by the literature, including themes relating to the role of significant relationships in initiating and supporting ongoing desistance as well as identity and behavioral changes of the desistance process. After the initial coding, I reviewed the transcripts again, revised my coding schematic, and applied it to the data. I looked for patterns that were occurring over time within and between respondents and mapped them using a visual display described by Saldana (2013). I mapped three main categories of codes and indicated the pathways between them. I began to see patterns that distinguished primary from secondary desistance. I noted the turning points and the aspects of significant relationships that facilitated respondents' capacity to engage in these phases. I reviewed my coding strategy and organized text segments into an interpretive schematic, utilizing tables that grouped relational factors associated with the desistance process.

Ethical Concerns

This section includes: (1) risks and protections of informed consent; (2) risks and protections of privacy; (3) risks and protections of harm; (4) benefits of participation; and (5) effects of MI on the research process. Reactivity and bias, trustworthiness of the data, and methodological challenges encountered during the data collection process are explored.

During the proposal process, I consulted with Heith Copes, PhD, Associate Professor, concerning the protocols for subject recruitment, risks, and protection from risks for this study. Dr. Copes is an expert researcher in interview-based studies of offenders. At the time of this study, he was a member of the University of Alabama's Institutional Review Board (IRB) and a member of my dissertation committee.

Risks to Informed Consent

Informed consent is an ethical challenge when potential respondents are members of cultural, racial, or medical minority groups but particularly when they have a criminal record and history. Men with such histories tend to be instinctively suspicious of anyone who appears to want something from them and in circumstances they may feel that they cannot refuse. Procedures designed to ensure full and informed consent of study respondents were detailed in the Sampling and Recruitment Procedures section.

Risks to Right to Privacy

Confidentiality is potentially problematic if a respondent were to disclose illegal activity for which he had not been adjudicated or if he reported that he engaged in child abuse. I specifically directed respondents in the informed consent process to withhold identifying information (such as dates, locations, and victims' names) about illegal activity. In this manner, were I subpoenaed, I would be unable to produce information that would increase the likelihood of a conviction. No respondents disclosed such behavior. The only exception is the reporting of child abuse, as researchers in the Commonwealth of Massachusetts are mandated reporters. The informed consent form addresses instances in which the researcher is mandated to report such acts. Additionally, respondents were informed that portions of audio tapes or transcripts could be shared with committee members or others involved in the research process and that I would utilize a confidential professional transcription service.

Digital interviews were uploaded to my password-protected personal computer and then deleted from the recorder. IRB study approval guidelines included that respondents were to sign the informed consent form with an "X" as a substitute for their names. The only paperwork containing respondent-identifying information was the list I tabulated of names and phone numbers left by potential respondents when they first called to express interest in the study. All other files and paperwork identify respondents by their pseudonyms only. Paper copies of forms, transcripts of the interviews, and other confidential data kept in my home office in a locked cabinet will be destroyed within 3 years of completion of the study. No identifying information will be included in any write-up or presentation of the data.

Risks of Harm

The potential harm to respondents includes threats to their legal and social standing and the possibility that the interview will cause distress. Respondents would be at legal risk if the following scenario were to occur: If during the interview, a respondent insisted on giving me detailed information about non-adjudicated offenses; if he were arrested after the interview; if he told police or prosecutors that he participated in this interview and that it includes incriminating information; if the respondent opted to go to trial instead of accepting a plea bargain; and if my records were subpoenaed. It was determined that this scenario was extremely unlikely to occur.

It is also possible that telling his story may induce emotional distress in a respondent: discussing his criminal past and relationships may cause him discomfort or agitation. Because their accounts were kept confidential throughout the project and anonymous when they were made public, risks to respondents' legal and social standing are minimal (H. Copes, personal communication, July 25, 2010). No one shared specific information with me about current or past non-adjudicated offenses.

Protecting study respondents from harm includes an analysis of the benefits and costs of participating (Miles & Huberman, 1994). Both of these aspects of engaging in the interview process were discussed with respondents during the consent process. In a recent study, inmates who had previously been interviewed for a research study concerning their criminal history were asked about their experiences with the interview process. They reported that the self-reflective aspect of the interview provided a number of benefits including: (1) an improvement in their outlook or behavior; (2) validation of their path to recovery; (3) the ability potentially to help others and to make amends; (4) an indication that the larger society does care about them; and (5) they hoped that changes to the CJ system could be brought about as a result of the research. Without exception, respondents described the interview as being a positive experience and reported that they did not experience harm from participating in the interview (Copes, Hochstetler, & Brown, 2013). Presser (2002) contacted her respondents by phone after the interview to check for any ill effects. She indicated that none of her 28 respondents reported them.

Feelings of guilt or remorse and the desire to atone for perceived wrongdoing are often motives for participating in research that examines stigmatized or criminalized behavior (Curtis, 2010). It is also my experience that reformed violent offenders often wish to make amends and cannot do so directly. This appeared to be the case for my respondents, many of whom engaged in volunteer work despite being unemployed and barely managing themselves. Participation in research is an indirect means with which to address damage they caused. For example, E refused my offer of the $25 remuneration until I suggested he could donate it. Potential benefits to those participating in this study also included having their prosocial narrative validated and improving their understanding of their desistance process.

Because this population has a high co-morbidity of substance abuse and mental illness, the risk of decompensation (the respondent becoming psychotic) was assessed on an ongoing basis as the interviews were conducted. There were no instances of respondents appearing agitated or psychotic but if these events had occurred, the interview would have been terminated and staff would have been notified to ensure that the respondent would be calmed. The interview would have been excluded from analysis as the decompensation would have negatively affected data quality.

The recruitment process was stopped during the spring of 2012 when my committee expressed concerns about the mental status of one of my respondents. The chair of my committee, Kathy Millstein, PhD, and I consulted with Gerald Koocher, PhD, ABPP, then Associate Provost and Professor of Psychology at Simmons College, an expert in the ethics of psychology practice and research, who clarified the issues specific to ethics and trustworthiness of the data and facilitated a comprehensive assessment of the impact of the interview before I proceeded. As most interviews took place at the location where respondents received services or volunteered, support staff was readily available if any respondent appeared to be suffering negative consequences from interview participation.

Reactivity and Bias

Although there is no consensus about how to define or measure the quality of qualitative research (Flick, 2007), threats to rigor and trustworthiness of the data and its analysis can be categorized broadly as (1) reactivity, the potentially distorting effects of the presence of the researcher; (2) researcher bias, viewing data through preconceived opinions or becoming emotionally too close or too far from respondents; and (3) respondent bias, deliberate withholding of information or lying to present an inaccurate presentation (Padgett, 1998). The "cure" for researcher bias is not to eliminate it but instead to make it transparent.

Researcher bias includes ways in which the researcher might inadvertently encourage the respondent to answer in a particular manner, thereby tainting the data and results. My bias in approaching this study was that I did not seek to confirm if relationships can have a positive impact on reducing violent behavior as based on the literature and my own practice experience, I know this to be true. Instead I was seeking to understand the ways in which they can create a positive impact. My ideas about the process that facilitates this outcome were described in the theoretical framework. I approached my respondents and the data with a healthy curiosity and expectation that I would learn more about aspects of the desistance process and other contributors to desistance related to significant relationships.

The interview protocol and study forms were evaluated by my committee and the IRB to ensure fair and unbiased language, thereby reducing reactivity and bias. Potential interviewer obstacles include my being a different gender and SES than my respondents and most often, a different race. Additionally, I do not share the vulnerabilities of my respondents in that I do not have a criminal record and have never been incarcerated. However, Weiss (1994) stated that if the interviewer is of higher societal rank than the respondent, it generally does not cause difficulty. I also found this to be true.

Respondent behavior is a particular issue with this population given its characterological propensity for prevarication (Yochelson & Samenow, 1985). Additionally, veracity of reports is a special concern when asking about retrospective accounts of stigmatized and sanctioned behaviors

(Bernasco, 2010) in which case, tendencies toward the use of exaggeration, minimization, distortion, justification, neutralization, denial, and preservation of favorable self-images become prominent (Brookman, 2010). Validity threats with this population include: (1) misinformation: the respondent does not have access to the requested information; (2) misunderstanding: both researcher and respondent are unaware of a mutual misunderstanding, often occurring as a result of "mismatching reference frames" (p.17); and (3) misleading: knowingly returning an incorrect answer (Elffers, 2010).

As a result of these concerns, many researchers recommend obtaining data from additional sources to compare with respondents' self-reports (Elffers, 2010; Lindegaard 2010). However, Miller (2010) stated that interviewers' socioemotional style including whether they are more personable or formal in their approach plays an important role in the accuracy and adequacy of responses. An open interview style is necessary. And Brookman (2010) declared, "the further one moves from observable, factual events towards internal thoughts and perceptions, the less feasible and desirable validation becomes" (p. 95). Therefore, Curtis (2010) stated that it is possible to collect reliable self-report information from respondents who have engaged in behavior that stigmatizes and marginalizes them and that "more often than not they tell the truth" (p. 152). He said that researchers often get far more cooperation than they expect.

Trustworthiness of the Data

The goal of rigor in qualitative research is to ensure that findings are representative of respondents' experiences, credible interpretations produce authentic, relevant findings (Padgett, 1998). External validity involves transferability—the ability of readers to apply the findings to their situations (Merriam & Associates, 2002). Additionally, social work research in particular concerns itself with the formulation of study-based implications for policy and practice (Padgett, 1998).

Of Padgett (1998)'s six most common methods to enhance study rigor and trustworthiness: (1) prolonged engagement; (2) triangulation; (3) peer debriefing and support; (4) member checking; (5) negative case analysis; and (6) an audit trail, I utilized four: triangulation, peer debriefing and support, negative case analysis, and an audit trail. I did not utilize prolonged engagement or member checking. Prolonged engagement was not feasible due to study design. I chose not to engage in member checking during analysis and writing up of the dissertation due to logistical issues (i.e., being unable to find respondents, literacy concerns).

Padgett (1998) detailed five types of triangulation: theory, methodological, observer, data, and interdisciplinary. This study utilized two: theory and interdisciplinary triangulation. Multiple theories were combined to produce the conceptual framework of the study. Although I was the lone researcher and thus did not collaborate with anyone else, my committee was composed of two social workers, two criminologists, and a community advisor who meets the study criteria. The chair of my committee read drafts of the codebook and portions of the data. She also consulted with Gerald Koocher, PhD, ABPP, then Associate Provost and Professor of Psychology at Simmons College and myself concerning issues related to the mental health status of my respondents. I chose not to engage in data triangulation due to ethical concerns.

I utilized my consultant, Laurie Pearlman, PhD, for debriefing and support throughout the data collection and analysis period. I read the transcripts carefully to ascertain any outlier responses or cases and to discover meanings other than those I had originally found. The audit trail for this study included a contact summary form completed after each interview, descriptive and reflective notes, analytic memos, iterations of the proposal, notes of committee meetings, email trails between me and committee members, and notes of a consult about ethical issues that arose during the interview process.

Methodological Challenges

As recruitment and sampling progressed, I found that some of my original assumptions about my ideal sample were challenged by the vagaries of snowball and convenience sampling and a difficult-to-access study population with multiple vulnerabilities. The large proportion of respondents with substance abuse, mental illness, and HIV disease was a product of the decision to recruit respondents through substance abuse and ex-offender treatment organizations. And as sampling progressed, adjustments to study protocols became necessary. Once I realized the literacy level of many of the study respondents, care was taken to ensure respondents understood the consent process. Inclusionary and exclusionary criteria were also changed during the recruitment process including length of time in the community, type of history of violence, and residence at sober houses.

The majority of study respondents did not read or write well so I approached the consent process carefully. I attempted to gauge the respondent's literacy by informal conversation prior to beginning the interview. If I thought he did not read well enough to understand the written version of the form (prepared at a seventh grade reading level as IRB approval mandated), I went over it verbally while he scanned so it would appear as if I were discussing items as he was reading. When I started to do this with respondents whose literacy was adequate to read the form, they would tell me it was not necessary. I would then answer any questions they asked.

The original inclusionary criteria for the sample group targeted men who had led a violence-free lifestyle for at least 5 years but had histories of serious acts of violence and multiple incarcerations. However, many of the respondents who participated in the study had not been violence-free or out of prison for the original length of time I had planned. Two primary factors affected the decision to include respondents with less time in desistance: accessing the sample through treatment organizations serving clients starting their desistance process and respondents not being truthful during the telephone screening.

The amount of time respondents reported being completely crime-free, violence-free, or out of prison varied from several months to over 10 years. Three respondents reported having been non-violent for 3 years or released from prison less than 5 years ago. Five respondents reported less than 1 year completely crime-free; they were newly sober and their coping skills were still being solidified. After consultation with my committee, I decided to include those respondents with less time in desistance due to the reliance on treatment organizations as the recruiting mechanism.

I had also wanted to exclude men who were currently on probation or parole and who were residents of halfway or sober houses. I believed that the structure provided by each of these entities might become confounding factors during data analysis, making it difficult to differentiate the impact of the external structures from respondents' internal desistance process. I ultimately maintained the exclusions related to CJ system status (probation, parole, or halfway house residence) due to increasing respondents' vulnerability. However, my first respondent and my recruiter were residents of an HIV sober house. The support of that program was consistent with the mechanisms I found in significant relationships. As a result of including those residing in treatment facilities, I was able to study the impact of HIV disease. I believe the incorporation of this factor enhances the research because HIV disease and substance abuse so often co-occur with violent behavior.

Two of the respondents lied during the telephone screening when asked about the length of time since they had been released from prison. It was only during the interview did I learn that they had been violence-free for less than 5 years. In consultation with my committee, I decided to include those interviews. After the inclusionary criteria was changed, when I was told during the telephone screening that a potential respondent had been violence-free or released from prison less than 5 years ago, I accepted him as a respondent.

It was also my original intention to interview men who had long histories of violence due to my assumption that those who commit one violent offense or several less serious ones could more easily establish desistance. The respondent group ended up being about evenly divided: six having a long criminal history and five being one time or less serious offenders. However, I did not find my assumption about desistance to be true. For example, the respondent with the least serious crime and shortest prison sentence was homeless, jobless, and mentally ill. Therefore, in retrospect, I think it was a benefit to have included a full range of violent offenders.

References

Bernasco, W. (2010). Preface. In W. Bernasco (Ed.), *Offenders on offending: Learning about crime from criminals* (pp. xxi–xxii). Devon, UK: Willan Publishing.

Copes, H., Hochstetler, A., & Brown, A. (2013). Ethical issues in inmate research: Inmates' perceptions of the benefits and harms of prison interviews. *Field Methods, 25*, 182–196.

Flick, U. (2007). *Designing qualitative research*. Los Angeles: Sage Publications.

Jacques, S., & Wright, R. (2010). Apprehending criminals: The impact of law on offender-based research. In W. Bernasco (Ed.), *Offenders on offending: Learning about crime from criminals* (pp. 23–48). Devon, UK: Willan Publishing.

Loeber, R., Pardini, D. A., Stouthamer-Loeber, M., & Raine, A. (2007). Do cognitive, physiological risk, and promotive factors predict desistance from delinquency in males? *Development and Psychopathology, 19*, 867–887.

Merriam, S. B., & Associates. (2002). *Qualitative research in practice: Examples for discussion and analysis*. San Francisco: Jossey-Bass.

Miles, M. B., & Huberman, A. M. (1994). *Qualitative data analysis: An expanded sourcebook* (2nd ed.). Thousand Oaks, CA: Sage Publications.

© The Editor(s) (if applicable) and The Author(s) 2016

D.H. Benveniste, *Changing Substance Abuse and Criminal Behavior Through Therapeutic Relationships*, DOI 10.1057/978-1-137-53039-4

Miller, J. (2010). The impact of gender interviewing 'offenders on offending'. In W. Bernasco (Ed.), *Offenders on offending: Learning about crime from criminals* (pp. 161–183). Devon, UK: Willan Publishing.

Moffitt, T. E. (1993). "Life-course persistent" and "adolescent-limited" antisocial behavior: A developmental taxonomy. *Psychological Review, 100*, 674–701.

Presser, L. (2002). Stories of violent men: Discursive construction of offender identities. Doctoral dissertation. Retrieved from Proquest Dissertation Abstracts International. (UMI number: 3060334.)

Soothill, K., Fitzpatrick, C., & Francis, B. (2009). *Understanding criminal careers*. Devon, UK: Willan Publishing.

Tewksbury, R., Dabney, D. A., & Copes, H. (2010). The prominence of qualitative research in criminology and criminal justice scholarship. *Journal of Criminal Justice Education, 21*, 391–411.

Weiss, R. S. (1994). *Learning from strangers: The art and method of qualitative interview studies*. New York: The Free Press.

Yochelson, S., & Samenow, S. E. (1985). *The criminal personality: The change process*. Northvale, NJ: Jason Aronson.

Index

© The Editor(s) (if applicable) and The Author(s) 2016
D.H. Benveniste, *Changing Substance Abuse and Criminal Behavior Through Therapeutic Relationships*, DOI 10.1057/978-1-137-53039-4

M

N

O

P

W

Printed by Printforce, the Netherlands